N

A

I

THE PREGNANT TEEN-AGER

A Medical, Educational, and Social Analysis

(Second Printing)

THE PREGNANT
TEEN-AGER

A Medical, Educational, and Social Analysis

By

HOWARD J. OSOFSKY, M.D.

Associate Professor of Obstetrics & Gynecology
State University of New York
Upstate Medical Center
Syracuse, New York

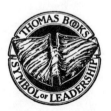

CHARLES C THOMAS • PUBLISHER
Springfield • Illinois • U.S.A.

Published and Distributed Throughout the World by
CHARLES C THOMAS • PUBLISHER
BANNERSTONE HOUSE
301–327 East Lawrence, Springfield, Illinois, U.S.A.
NATCHEZ PLANTATION HOUSE
735 North Atlantic Boulevard, Fort Lauderdale, Florida, U.S.A.

ISBN 0-398-01434-5

Library of Congress Catalog Card Number: 68–9391

First Printing, 1968
Second Printing, 1972

With THOMAS BOOKS *careful attention is given to all details of
manufacturing and design. It is the Publisher's desire to present books
that are satisfactory as to their physical qualities and artistic possibilities
and appropriate for their particular use.* THOMAS BOOKS *will be true
to those laws of quality that assure a good name and good will.*

Printed in the United States of America
N-1

PREFACE

The problems of pregnant teen-agers are receiving an increased amount of emphasis both in the United States and abroad. This emphasis relates to several factors. First of all, both the actual numbers and relative incidence of such pregnancies have been increasing at a rapid rate. For example, in 1965, the year for which the latest complete statistics are available, 591,000 teen-agers were reported to have given birth in this country (U.S. Department of Health, Education and Welfare, 1968).

But it is not only the actual number of teen-age pregnancies which has led to the growth of concern; it is accompanying factors. Forty percent, or 129,000 of the above-cited teen-age pregnancies, were delivered out of wedlock. Another 120,000 were conceived out of wedlock. These figures do not include the large number of out-of-wedlock pregnancies which are kept from the statistics because of concealment or abortion. Further, even where marriage was present, often there were problems related to the very young age of the partners—or to the situation of the marriage having been forced because of the existent pregnancy.

Pregnancy in the young provokes many questions which need to be asked. There is concern about the behavior and principles of the involved teen-agers and of teen-agers in general. There is also concern because of the appreciable financial costs of teen-age pregnancies to the community. Marked increases have been required in the amount of financial assistance provided for the mothers and their surviving infants. Legislators and taxpayers alike have demonstrated their concern over the mounting cost of this support.

Along with the growing awareness of the size and financial components of the problem, at least some recognition has been given to the relative paucity of services which is at present avail-

v

able to this group of medically and socioeconomically high-risk individuals. As will be discussed in detail, in most areas within the United States, little meaningful help is available to teen-agers during pregnancy, and even less help has been available to assist the girls in making a meaningful re-entry into society. Medical care, social service counseling, and educational opportunities have all been woefully inadequate. For many teen-agers, pregnancy has resulted in the ending of all ambitions, goals, and plans for the future. For the girls, for their offspring, and for society in general, such results of teen-age pregnancy have markedly worrisome, long-range implications.

My personal involvement with the problems of pregnant teen-agers has been intense for a variety of reasons. As a physician and medical educator, I first became concerned with the morbidity and mortality figures for this group. I later became concerned with the developmental prognosis of the infants born to pregnant teen-agers. I have repeatedly found myself wondering how one can reach out to these individuals who are at major risk medically, and how one can meaningfully improve the anticipated outcome for this high-risk group of individuals.

As I have become more concerned with the medical problems of this particular group, other humanistic considerations have also assumed increasingly greater proportions. I have become aware, not only of the major medical problems facing pregnant teen-agers, but of the social and educational problems as well. I have come to realize that regardless of one's point of view, the pregnant teen-ager is indeed an individual at high risk. In this book, I hope to share with the reader the reasons which have led me to such conclusions, and some possible solutions to the problems involved.

Since October 1965, I have served as medical director of the Y-MED (Young Mothers Educational Development) Program in Syracuse, New York. This program, which operates under the sponsorship of the Syracuse Board of Education, the Onondaga County Department of Health, and the State University of New York, Upstate Medical Center at Syracuse, has attempted, under one roof, with a day-care center philosophy, to provide meaningful medical, educational, and social service facilities for pregnant teen-agers. The program is open to all girls, regardless of the complexity and severity of their needs. Since its inception, no girl who has been desirous of entering the program has been turned away. The program is client-centered; the staff has attempted to operate on a truly interdisciplinary basis, and has at all times a respectful, noncondescending orientation towards the girls and their needs.

Approximately 225 girls have begun care at this facility. One hundred have undergone delivery, and almost all of these girls are still receiving some degree of support through the program facilities. This book will not specifically deal with the Y-MED program. Nor will it deal with the exciting results which are emanating from the program. Any reader who is interested in the philosophy, the operation, and results of the program is referred to available publications (Braen, 1968; Osofsky, 1967a, 1968a, 1968b). I do, however, allude to our results where they are of pertinence in shedding light upon some questions to be raised in later sections of the book.

Another important reason for discussing the program is that my association with the Y-MED program, its personnel, and the girls involved as patients, clients, and students, has been a very meaningful one. I truly believe that the experience has resulted in an intense personal growth and in an often-painful introspective re-evaluation of my own thinking. Two years ago I was a more traditional physician, and in the framework of my present thinking, a more "bigoted individual." I could not at that time have realized the staggering problems facing pregnant teen-agers. I had often wondered why medical care was so poor for these individuals. I did not fully realize the role which physicians and medical personnel played in determining the inadequacy of care. As a physician, I had little awareness of the policies of social service departments, welfare agencies, boards of education, law enforcement agencies, and a multitude of other official and unofficial community resources. I was aware of some of the motivational difficulties experienced by this group. I was little aware of the large burden of guilt which society must assume because of its contribution to the already existent problems of pregnant teen-agers.

The views expressed are not necessarily those of the official agencies sponsoring the Y-MED program. Nor will they represent the views of all the staff members of the program. Obviously, my ideas have been influenced by the probing questions and even painful suggestions of my professional colleagues and close friends within the program. Often, my opinions will have been further influenced by the comments and the problems of individual girls, and by my successful, or unsuccessful, attempts to deal with these problems. But, by necessity, many of the conclusions will be those which have come to make sense for me as an individual.

It is my conviction that much factual information is available concerning pregnant teen-agers. Some of this information I hope to share. The book will not, however, be confined to factual information alone. As a human being, I feel far too strongly about some of the issues and some of the injustices which I perceive to exist, not to share these with the reader. I mention these feelings in advance for they will appear in various sections of the book. I do not apologize for including such subjective ideas. Society in general and those individuals responsible for services to pregnant teen-agers are faced with real problems. If better care is to be given, a more meaningful and realistic interpretation must be made concerning what is now available and what changes should be made within the near future.

HOWARD J. OSOFSKY

ACKNOWLEDGMENTS

As is true of most authors, I sincerely feel a debt of gratitude to many persons who have directly and indirectly made this book possible. Obviously, not all of them can be singled out. However, some of them have assumed such a vital and direct role in my own growth and development that I would feel remiss if I did not at least mention them. Dr. Robert Austin, Dr. Bernard Braen, Mr. Robert DiFlorio, Dr. John Hagen, Dr. Robert Long, and Mrs. Peggy W. Wood have all served as my trusted colleagues and mentors during the past two years. The remainder of the staff at Y-MED will not be singled out by name. However, I could cite each individual member. Each, in his unique manner, has contributed to my own evolvement and to my own present day thinking. Dr. David Bigwood, Onondaga County Commissioner of Health; Dr. Virginia Harris, Director of Maternal and Child Welfare for Onondaga County; Dr. Franklyn Barry, Syracuse Superintendent of Schools; Mr. Henry Balmer, Director of Special Projects for the Syracuse Board of Education; and Dr. George Murdock, Commissioner of School Health for the Syracuse Board of Education, should all be singled out. With these individuals, during the past two years, I have worked hard and occasionally fought hard; from all of them I have learned much concerning the problems of the dedicated community servant and his overwhelming difficulties in improving the quality of available care. Perhaps, most of all, I should thank the 225 girls who have to the present time attended the Y-MED program. To varying extents, they have allowed me to share some of their successes, their problems, and their real hurts. They have acted both as my mentors and my tormentors. They have assisted in my own growth and in my capacity to give. I would also like to thank Miss Joanne Golas,

Miss Marjorie Gillette, and Mrs. Edith Brigham. These fine secretaries have worked laboriously with me; without their efforts, the completion of this work would have been impossible.

Three people should be singled out for special appreciation. Mrs. Karen DeCrow has devoted many hours to editing the final draft of this manuscript. Her advice and assistance have been invaluable to its preparation. The Chairman of the Department of Obstetrics and Gynecology at the Upstate Medical Center, Dr. Robert E. L. Nesbitt, Jr., has been of major help to me. In my four years of association with him, he has constantly encouraged me and aided my development. The departmental resources have always been made available; his mature and inciteful wisdom have been extremely important in my own progress and in the growth of programs with which I have been associated. My wife, Joy D. Osofsky, should also be singled out, and I have saved this for last. I know that most authors acknowledge a debt of appreciation to their wives. For me, this debt is a special one. Often, my work has resulted in sixteen-hour days and seven-day weeks. Her understanding and the depth of her own interests have allowed for such commitment on my part. To her, to the others mentioned, and to those not singled out by name, I express sincere appreciation. To a great extent, whatever small accomplishment I may make is related to their efforts and to their relationships with me.

H.J.O.

CONTENTS

THE PREGNANT TEEN-AGER

A Medical, Educational, and Social Analysis

I

THE SCOPE OF THE PROBLEM

The pregnant teen-ager belongs to several subgroups. It is difficult for the researcher to identify which of these is the most significant, for all are important.

The pregnant teen-ager is not only young and female, but she has deviated from accepted social norms (premarital intercourse may be prevalent, but only lip service is paid to its possible appropriateness in American life); and in a majority of reported cases, she is poor and nonwhite. Although a popular misconception exists that the poor and especially the nonwhite accept illegitimate births, this author thinks, on the basis of research and professional experience, that such is not the case: in a society where unwed mothers are looked down on, all socioeconomic and racial groups have negative attitudes toward illegitimate pregnancies. Richer persons simply have more effective means of dealing with contraception, the concealment or termination of unwanted pregnancy, and adoption.

The problems of the pregnant teen-ager are complex. This book divides them in the following way: medical, social service, and educational. The last two chapters deal with sex education, contraception, and abortion.

Teen-agers of any description represent members of multiple subclasses, dependent upon parental background, ethnic origin, socioeconomic status, and the community where they live, just to mention a few of the possible categories. A black teen-ager in Harlem has a very different existence from that of an affluent, white teen-ager in Grosse Pointe. Both may be going through physiologic and psychologic storms of adolescence. Yet these upheavals represent only part of their total existence. The black youth in Harlem, except for age, bears more similarity to other

3

inner-city adolescents and to adult members of the Harlem community than he does to the adolescent in Grosse Pointe. His medical problems, nutritional deficiencies, educational experiences, and economic opportunities have a greater kinship to others in lower socioeconomic urban areas, and especially to black groups in these areas, than they do to white affluent suburbanites. Yet, if one were to discuss physiologic and psychologic developmental changes, or if one were to look at patterns of educational progress, one would be justified in making comparisons with teen-agers from a different environmental background and with very different potential opportunities. Thus, only after knowing the questions to be raised can one make the decision as to which is the appropriate group for comparison. To answer certain questions, it is appropriate to make comparisons with peer groups of different backgrounds. Other areas of investigation should use as comparison groups those from similar ethnic backgrounds, regardless of age. In some studies, sex is the crucial comparison factor.

Since 40 percent of all out-of-wedlock pregnancies are reported as occurring among teen-agers (Vincent, 1961), and since a high percentage of pregnancies occurring among teen-agers are conceived out of wedlock, it is important to view some of the problems of pregnant teen-agers within the context of the problems of the female who is pregnant out of wedlock.

Because 60 percent of reported out-of-wedlock pregnancies occur among members of the nonwhite population, some of the special problems which are related to racial background must be considered in understanding the problems of the pregnant teen-ager. Knowing that nationally 50 percent of the children receiving aid to dependent children have been delivered out of wedlock (Tuttle, 1962), it becomes important to look at teen-age pregnancy, in part, in relationship to some of the problems of poverty, and, often, in relationship to the problems of urban poverty. Since such pregnancy represents the number one cause of school dropout among females (Stine, 1964), and since many of these dropouts occur within inner-city schools, it becomes important to look at some of the educational problems connected with teen-age pregnancy. The group can again be subdivided on medical grounds, comparing the medical complications of individuals with different backgrounds, and how they relate to age, nutrition, ethnic origin, and socioeconomic status.

Another category useful for study is that of adolescence itself. Along with traditional adolescent upheavals, the changing patterns which are at present occurring in adolescent life—including alterations in social and sexual attitudes—obviously relate to the problems of teen-age pregnancy. What clearly emerges, therefore, is an intricate picture of the pregnant adolescent.

THE TEEN-AGER AS OUT-OF-WEDLOCK MOTHER

Both in the United States and abroad, the number of out-of-wedlock pregnancies has been dramatically increasing, not only in absolute numbers, but as a percentage of the total number of delivered live births as well. The figures available from New York City demonstrate this trend. In New York, in 1946, it was estimated that 3 percent of all pregnancies were delivered out of wedlock; by 1959, this figure had reached 8 percent; and by 1963, 11 percent of all reported pregnancies were listed as being delivered out of wedlock (Rashbaum, 1963). Nationally, the direction of the figure is similar although the exact percentages are slightly different.

In the United States, in 1938, 87,900 pregnancies were reported as occurring among unwed mothers, comprising 3.6 percent of the total number of live births for that year. By 1960, the figure had reached approximately 225,000 and represented 5.2 percent of that year's births (Vincent, 1961). For 1965, the figure had grown to 291,000—or 7.7 percent of the total births (U.S. Department of Health, Education, and Welfare, 1968). In other countries the reported trends parallel those in this country. In England, for example, in 1961 it was estimated that one out of 20 children was born illegitimately, one in eight was conceived out of marriage, and one in four mothers conceived their first born offspring before marriage (*Lancet* editorial, 1961). The magnitude of the figures is indeed striking.

Large as these percentages are, however, it must be remembered that the numbers of out-of-wedlock pregnancies which

The Pregnant Teen-Ager

TABLE I

OUT OF WEDLOCK LIVE BIRTHS AND TOTAL LIVE BIRTHS
IN THE UNITED STATES BY YEAR

Year	Number of Live Births	Number of Out of Wedlock Live Births	Out of Wedlock Pregnancies as Percent of the Total
1938	2,286,962	87,900	3.0%
1940	2,360,399	89,500	3.6%
1945	2,735,456	117,400	4.6%
1950	3,554,149	141,600	3.9%
1955	4,047,295	183,300	4.5%
1960	4,257,850	224,300	5.2%
1965	3,760,358	291,100	7.8%

Abstracted from Department of Health, Education and Welfare Vital Statistics Reports

are reported each year cannot fully portray the actual number of such pregnancies which are occurring. Many pregnancies, which should be classified as out of wedlock, escape inclusion in the reports. For example, when women are legally married, but become pregnant extramaritally, these pregnancies are not listed as occurring out of wedlock. Similarly, offspring delivered to a legally separated woman who is not living with her husband, and whose husband is not responsible for the pregnancy, still are not classified routinely on birth certificate records as out of wedlock. Frequently, "hasty marriages" are performed after conception in order to legalize the birth of the future offspring. Such marriages may terminate in planned divorces following childbirth, but, again, the pregnancies are not designated as occurring out of wedlock. And, of course, there are numerous instances where records are either inadequately kept or deliberately falsified in order to protect the pregnant woman. Thus, the reported figures, high as they are, do not take into account the total number of pregnancies delivered out of wedlock. If more accurate data could be obtained, the figures would be much higher.

However, even if it were possible somehow to accurately distinguish from birth records the percentage of infants conceived outside of marriage, a major source of out-of-wedlock conceptions would still remain unreported. Since the records could only report infant deliveries, the large number of out-of-wedlock pregnancies which are terminated by illegal abortion would not be considered. There are no accurate figures concerning illegal abortion. Most estimates have placed the numbers at between 1,000,000 and 2,000,000 annually in the United States (NOW, 1967; Roemer, 1967). However, other estimates have ranged from reports of as low as several hundred thousand to reports which suggest that for every child delivered in this country each year, another pregnancy is aborted illegally. Even if the true figures do not approach this upper estimate of 4,500,000, and even if 1,000,000 is a closer estimate of the number, the magnitude of the numbers is still most impressive. The annual number of abortions appears to dwarf the number of live births which are reported as occurring out of wedlock.

Obviously, not all illegal abortions are performed upon women conceiving extramaritally. A significant number occur to women who are married, but not desirous of that pregnancy. Yet few would deny that a high number of illegal abortions are performed upon women who are either not married or who are married to someone other than the man who sired the pregnancy. The social, educational, and even medical problems of the women who are pregnant out of wedlock and who obtain illegal abortions are considerably different from the problems which pertain to the women who are pregnant out of wedlock but who carry their pregnancies to term.

Teen-agers, of course, do not account for all of the out-of-wedlock pregnancies which occur annually. If one looks at the figures comparing percentage increases in reported out-of-wedlock pregnancies, the greatest proportional increase has occurred in the group of women age 25 and above. However, these women still contribute a relatively small percentage of the total number of infants born out of wedlock.

Teen-agers, on the other hand, contribute a disproportionately high percentage of such infants. It is estimated that approximately 40 percent of all illegitimate pregnancies occur in females under the age of 20. In 1965, in the United States,

TABLE II

OUT OF WEDLOCK LIVE BIRTHS—BY AGE OF MOTHER—FOR 1965
IN THE UNITED STATES

Age of Mother	Number of Out-of-Wedlock Births
Under Age 15	6,100
Age 15—19	123,000
Age 20—24	90,600
Age 25—29	36,800
Age 30—34	19,600
Age 35 and older	15,000

Abstracted from Department of Health, Education and Welfare Vital Statistics
Reports

129,000 of the 291,000 reported out-of-wedlock pregnancies
occurred in women under the age of 20. Of further interest, not
only do teen-agers account for a high percentage of reported
out-of-wedlock pregnancies, but a considerable number of teen-
age pregnancies are conceived out of wedlock.

TABLE III

MARRIED AND OUT-OF-WEDLOCK LIVE BIRTHS BY AGE OF MOTHER
FOR 1965 IN THE UNITED STATES

Mother's Age	Married Live Births	Out-of-Wedlock Live Births	Total Live Births
Under Age 15	1,668	6,100	7,768
Age 15—19	467,894	123,000	590,894
Age 20—24	1,246,750	90,600	1,337,350
Age 25—29	888,932	36,800	925,732
Age 30—34	509,776	19,600	529,376
Age 35 and older	354,238	15,000	369,238

Abstracted from Department of Health, Education and Welfare Vital Statistics
Reports

The figures concerning teen-age marriage and teen-age pregnancy tend to bear out this statement quite clearly. The absolute
number of teen-age marriages has been steadily rising throughout the United States, and the percentage of marriages occurring
between two teen-agers has been increasing at a proportionally

faster rate than marriages in general among older population groups. In 1949, 33 percent of couples marrying were teen-agers. By 1959, the percentage had risen to 39 percent (Wallace, 1965). The average age for couples marrying has decreased both for males and for females. Associated with these increasing numbers of teen-age marriages is a high incidence of marital complications. The highest rate of divorce occurs among couples married in their teens. The divorce rate of this group is three to four times higher than that for couples who marry at a later age (Rankin, 1964). Accompanying the earlier age of marriage has been an increasing incidence of teen-age pregnancy, with the accompanying alteration in job and educational expectation which may follow for either or both parents. In 1950, 27 percent of first born babies were delivered to mothers who were in their teens. In 1959, the proportion had increased to 36 percent; by 1965, it had reached 39 percent of all first born infants delivered in that year (U.S. Department of Health, Education and Welfare, 1968; Wallace, 1965).

One of the major problems, which often goes unconsidered, is that the high incidence of teen-age pregnancies often is the etiologic cause of, rather than the result of, teen-age marriage. As has previously been mentioned in the statistics concerning England, one out of four first born pregnancies is conceived prior to marriage. These statistics relate to all first born pregnancies, regardless of maternal age. Recent figures, reported from California, indicate that among teen-agers this figure is considerably higher. The California figures indicate that approximately 50 percent of marriages between two high school students in that state involve an already conceived pregnancy (Landis, 1964). Thus, one clearly sees an important, and somewhat disconcerting, fact. The number of first born babies delivered to teen-agers is increasing at a considerably more rapid rate than the number of first born deliveries to other age groups in the population; of this growing number, a considerable percentage have been conceived out of wedlock. For reasons previously mentioned, this large number of teen-age pregnancies, conceived out of wedlock, but followed by marriage, does not get included in the figures reporting teen-age out-of-wedlock pregnancies. Yet, in spite of this exclusion, teen-age pregnancies account for 40 percent of all reported out-of-wedlock pregnancies.

When one looks at girls who are pregnant in the early teens, the figures are even more striking: 2.1 percent of all out-of-wedlock pregnancies occur in individuals who are younger than 15 years of age. When one studies mothers who are younger than 15 years of age as a group, however, one discovers that 88.7 percent of all their pregnancies have been conceived out of wedlock (Pakter, 1961a). Thus the general problem clearly emerges. Teen-agers account for a considerable proportion of the known out-of-wedlock pregnancies. Obviously, the figures are even more striking in the younger teens than they are in females approaching 20. And, again, none of these figures include the pregnancies which are somehow hidden or aborted. Therefore, one must consider many of the teen-age mothers as a particular subgroup of the general category of out-of-wedlock mothers.

THE PREGNANT TEEN-AGER AS MEMBER OF THE POOR

Another categorization, which is appropriate in looking at the problems of the pregnant teen-ager, is that of financial background. Not all pregnant teen-agers are poor, just as not all women who become pregnant out of wedlock or under other difficult circumstances are poor. Illegitimate and unwanted pregnancies occur to members of all economic classes, but they are particularly noticeable and are considered particularly prevalent among the poor. It is, however, difficult to gain an unbiased estimate of the exact representation of varying financial backgrounds among teen-age girls who become pregnant, especially among those who become pregnant out of wedlock.

There are many reasons for this difficulty. They all can be categorized under the statement: the poor are less able to control their own fate. They have neither the money, nor the political power, nor the social savvy, to incorporate their own needs and desires into the mainstream of acceptable society. Individuals from the middle and upper socioeconomic class are often better able to conceal their pregnancies, and even to conceal the status of illegitimacy from birth certificate records. The incidence of hasty or forced marriage may also vary on the basis of socioeconomic class.

But, one incalculable set of circumstances most biases the accuracy of data collection. Women from the middle and upper socioeconomic class are more likely to obtain illegal abortions because of both greater social mobility and available money. Kinsey's data (1958) demonstrates that the actual obtaining of abortions is related to socioeconomic class. He estimates that the overwhelming percentage of abortions in the United States are obtained by white women; relatively few are obtained by nonwhite women. Obviously, this racial breakdown has socioeconomic implications, since the majority of the nonwhite population is from the lower socioeconomic group.

Thus one sees a paradox which often becomes apparent when looking at the problems of teen-age and other pregnant individuals. Inequality of opportunity on the basis of socioeconomic and ethnic background results in a difference in methods available to solve problems. The well-to-do and ethnically favored groups are better able legally and extralegally to handle difficult problems. The poor and nonwhite members of the population do not have such solutions as part of their armamentarium. Yet the society which does not grant them equal opportunity criticizes and even legally punishes them for the problems which may stem from the existence of the inequality.

One of the social and legal issues which has created great unrest is that of the mounting financial cost to the community of out-of-wedlock pregnancy and aid to the surviving children. The majority of women pregnant out of wedlock and their surviving infants do not receive governmental financial support. It is estimated that fewer than 10 percent of the white and 16 percent of the nonwhite children who are delivered out of wedlock receive aid to dependent children (Vincent, 1961). However, because the annual number of reported out-of-wedlock pregnancies is already so large, and because the number is rising at such a rapid rate, the amount of assistance given to this relatively small percentage adds up to a large sum of money. Nationally, it is estimated that 50 percent of the children who receive aid to dependent children have been delivered out of wedlock (Tuttle, 1962). It is further estimated that social welfare costs for the average mother who becomes pregnant out of wedlock before the age of 20, and who requires assistance, is $100,000 during the remainder of her lifetime. Although the figure at first glance seems high, it has been further estimated that the average teen-ager, who becomes pregnant out of wedlock, carries her pregnancy to term, and requires welfare assistance, has an additional eight children during the course of her lifetime, all of whom may require some social welfare assistance. Further, this figure includes only direct social welfare payments, and does not include special educational and other indirect costs to the community, which will be discussed in later sections (Krantz, 1965).

Although the $100,000 figure seems plausible, considering the number of persons being cared for over a number of years, it is a considerable sum. The society might do well to reevaluate its dole system, which might be summarized as being "penny wise and pound foolish." If the cost of all programs to train for job skills, social abilities, and other assimilating techniques, were looked at with an eye to the alternative cost of supporting certain subgroups, we might have a social order not only more humanitarian, but more fiscally prudent.

Because of the mounting costs to the community related to out-of-wedlock pregnancies, the public has shown increasing concern. There have been recent attempts to tie strings to the assistance programs for unmarried mothers and their infants. Qualifications have been included in legislation mandating that these mothers seek future contraception, and education or work. Although one might severely question the constitutional and moral appropriateness of such legislation, its very consideration indicates the growing anxiety which the community cost for out-of-wedlock pregnancies has raised.

THE PREGNANT TEEN-AGER AS NONWHITE

The national statistics for reported out-of-wedlock pregnancies indicate that 60 percent occur among nonwhite females. The percentages, based upon age alone, do not appear to differ for pregnant teen-agers. Again, it is important to note that these figures are biased because of failure to account for illegal abortions, and that, if the figures were corrected by including the large number of abortions which occur annually, the ratio percentages for out-of-wedlock conceptions would more closely approximate the actual ethnic ratio percentages in the population. However, the fact remains that of the infants who are reported delivered out of wedlock annually in this country, the bulk are nonwhite.

When one takes nonwhite teen-age females as a group, and especially when one adds poverty and inner-city dwelling, as most often is the case, one faces special difficulties in the areas of medical care and prognosis, social service counseling, and educational opportunity. Where pregnancy compounds the inequality faced by nonwhite, poor, inner-city inhabitants, the difficulties are severe, and in some cases may be insurmountable. Therefore, it is important, even after one considers the reasons which lead to the disproportionately large number of nonwhite infants who are delivered out of wedlock, to look at some of the problems which exist for the mothers and for these infants, since such birth do occur, and the resultant problems do exist.

THE PREGNANT TEEN-AGER AS TEEN-AGER

One other major area must be considered if one is to adequately view the problems of pregnant teen-agers. This area is that of adolescence itself. In addition to being members of some of the previously described subgroups, pregnant teen-agers also represent adolescents with some of the special problems and difficulties which are unique to this stage of life (Blos, 1964; Erikson, 1961; Freud, 1958; Friedenberg, 1957; Naegele, 1961; Millman, 1965; Spiegel, 1958; Toussieng, 1965). In some cultures the marked psychological upheaval, which is observed in all areas of Western civilization, does not appear to exist (Benedict, 1938; Bettelheim, 1961; Eisenstadt, 1961, Mead, 1955; Whiting, 1953). In such societies, at the time of puberty, individuals

become members of adult society. They are then expected to
function as adults and are given not only adult responsibilities,
but adult privileges as well. The continued physiologic changes
which normally occur during the teen years are accepted much
as other physiologic changes, such as those which occur during
the forties and fifties when menses cease, are accepted. Teen-
agers, in such societies appear less rebellious and seem to accept
their new adult responsibilities with relative ease (Benedict,
1938; Mead, 1955; Whiting, 1953).

In modern Western culture there are practical reasons which
make it difficult to allow the teen-ager to be a fully-functioning
adult. The culture is advanced technologically. Occupations,
and especially the more sought after occupations, require years
of study and prior preparation. Males and females at puberty
are not educated enough to assume any of the top positions in
the community. Their training and education must continue,
and this continuation places the teen-ager in a role of dependence—dependence upon parents, teachers, and other authority
figures within the community. For most teen-agers, financial and,
at least in part, emotional dependence upon meaningful adults
remains for several years following puberty.

This dependence is responsible for some of the mixed feelings
which result from the teen-agers' striving for autonomy at the
same time he or she desires parental support and approval.
There are, however, other controls placed upon teen-agers in
modern day society of questionable meaning and necessity. For
obvious educational and technological reasons, teen-agers are
not in positions of economic or professional power. Yet society
requires teen-agers to behave in an adult manner, and to demonstrate mature attitudes. Irresponsibility and immature behavior
are condemned by the adult world. Yet autonomy and a respectful orientation from the adult world toward his individual strivings and attitudes are denied to the teen-ager. Not only is the
teen-ager dependent for sustenance and education upon the adult
world, but other meaningful decisions are made for him by the
adult world. Although teen-agers are expected to be part of armies,
they have no voice in deciding where and when wars should be
fought. Although teen-agers are expected to act with adult re-

sponsibility, they have no vote and, therefore, no real voice in community affairs and decision-making.

The full impact of adult ambivalence toward adolescent strivings can be noted in the area of sexual behavior. A confused and conflicted message is given to teen-agers. They, like adults, are living in a society which has experienced a revolution both in thought and action concerning sexual behavior. There has been a greater freedom in expression concerning sexual activity, as can be seen from the books of such authors as Kinsey (1943, 1958) and Masters and Johnson (1966), and from material which is shown daily in the mass media. Along with a freer discussion of sexual behavior, there has been a widespread belief that sexual standards and mores in general have become more relaxed. Adults and even church groups have voiced opinions that behaviors, formerly considered to be either immoral or sinful, are now acceptable in particular circumstances.

Along with a general relaxation of sexual standards, there has existed an already confused image of appropriate sexual behavior. It has long been felt appropriate by many adults for adolescent males to engage in premarital sexual behavior and intercourse. At the same time, at least until recently, the Victorian mores which guided attitudes in this country dictated the importance of virginity for the female at the time of marriage. A double standard was set up which could not easily be resolved for the individuals involved. At the present time, lip service is paid by adults to the appropriateness of reexamining these mores. Teen-agers have found themselves also involved in redefining acceptable sexual behavior.

There have been other uncertainties which have led to present day teen-age difficulty in dealing with sexual drives and behavior. The past fifty years have witnessed a marked upheaval in the delineation of social structure and support. Part of this upheaval is clearly exemplified by significant changes in the role of the family. There has been a general decline in family closeness, especially in that of the relationships of the extended family. Family supports, traditions, and dictates upon individual members have weakened considerably. At the same time that the role of the family in providing emotional support and pressure has declined, there has been an increase in other types of pressures. Population growth, automation of industry, scientific and technological advances, and availability of leisure time are examples of some of the changes, which in themselves have created new and different pressures. Travel and communication have both become more sophisticated. Individuals have been exposed to a wider variety of opinions and ideas, and have become aware of alternatives to their own thinking and backgrounds. In a localized subculture where each person knew every other person, certain types of attitudes and behaviors went unquestioned. With broader access to other values, the members now find occasion to question their mores.

Thus, a complex set of problems face the adolescent. Like adults, adolescents live in a faster, more technological, and more pressured world. Their families may not be as close knit as would have been true in their parents' teen-age experience; even their parents may offer less guidance and advice. They live in a world where expressed adult opinions concerning sexual behavior acknowledge a more permissive and liberal attitude. At the same time, particular parents still have difficulty discussing sexual attitudes and behavior with children, and relatively few schools have meaningful discussions of these topics. Further, as will be discussed in more detail at a later point, contraception, especially for the female, is neither discussed nor available.

Sexually, the adolescent is in a difficult position. In some societies, adolescents would be considered adults sexually as well as in other spheres of their lives. In our society, adolescents, already confused by their role in general, are further confused by the dictates of what may be considered appropriate sexual behavior. They are told to behave as adults and to consider themselves as adults. There are even adult hints which suggest freer sexual behavior; erotic sexual material is constantly at their disposal. Males are to some extent even encouraged to demonstrate their sexual prowess. Yet in the final analysis the adult society still puts taboos upon teen-age heterosexual behavior. Not only in attitudes toward contraception, but especially in attitudes toward premarital teen-age pregnancy, the adult world is considerably judgmental and punitive. There is much shame, pressure, and undesirable social stigma attached to premarital teen-age pregnancy. For teen-age girls, and to a lesser extent for teen-age boys, there is much difficulty, and even disgrace, involved with such pregnancy. The teen-ager is in a progressively more difficult rule. No longer a child, and yet not accepted as an adult, he is faced with taboos and restrictions, and at the same time increasing drives and encouragement toward at least a pseudotype of individual decision-making. The decisions, regardless of their direction, are difficult ones for the teen-ager to make.

Teen-age pregnancy can be classified and studied from a variety of points of view. The social problem of out-of-wedlock pregnancy is often a central focus. Poverty, with its resultant pressures for the individual and for the community at large, is a frequent area of concentration. Because such a high percentage of pregnancies which come to term occur in nonwhite members of the population, the difficulties which pregnancies create for nonwhite mothers must be considered as one part of the problem. The special problems of being a teen-ager, and especially, a teen-ager in a complex society which offers conflicting messages to adolescents, must also be inspected.

The multiple problems are difficult and interwoven; they have only been touched upon in the preceding paragraphs. In the coming sections, an attempt will be made to view in detail some of the specific problems which confront the pregnant teen-ager in the vital areas of medical care and prognosis, social service counseling, and educational opportunities.

II

THE MEDICAL PROBLEM

SOME GENERAL OBSTETRICAL CONCEPTS

A concern over the attainment of good health for all members of society is a fundamental concept in American life. Since the turn of the century, medical advances in the United States have resulted in a life expectancy increase of 25 years. Poliomyelitis has been virtually eradicated; tuberculosis has become less of a problem; infections are usually brought under control by antibiotics; hemorrhage is treated by blood. The list could go on indefinitely.

In obstetrics, the figures concerning childbirth are impressive. From 1930 to 1958, the number of maternal deaths per 10,000 live births decreased from 67 to 3.8 (Eastman, 1961). Similarly, though not quite so striking, the number of infants born dead per 1,000 live births (fetal death rate) decreased from 38.1 in 1926 to 22.4 in 1952, and to 17.1 in 1955; the number of infants dying during the first four weeks of life per 1,000 live births (neonatal death rate) decreased from 37.8 in 1925 to 19.8 in 1952 (Eastman, 1961; Nesbitt, 1957; U. S. Dept. of Health, Education and Welfare, 1968). The reasons for the progress during this period of time are numerous; among them are some of the dramatic advances in medical knowledge, including blood for transfusion, antibiotics for infection, and the improvement of prenatal care in general. Since the early 1950's, however, a considerable change has occurred in the overall picture. The fetal and neonatal death rates which had been improving at such a rapid rate began to level off. Whereas the fetal mortality rate had diminished by 6.8 per 1,000 live births between 1945 and 1955, the next ten years were marked by a fall of only .9 per 1,000 live births. The perinatal mortality slowdown is equally

18

striking; between 1955 and 1964, a total reduction of only 2.3 per 1,000 live births was noted (U. S. Dept. of Health, Education and Welfare, 1968). Had the United States' figures of the 1940's and 1950's continued to improve to the present time, this country would now favorably compare with other countries throughout the world. Instead, the figures in several other countries, especially those in Scandinavia, continue to be considerably better than those reported from this country (Chase, 1967). At present, there is little indication to suggest that a marked change will occur in the near future.

Because of the desire to further increase life expectancy and to decrease incapacity related to illness, the past 20 years have been marked by changing concepts in obstetrical and neonatal care. Although basic philosophies have differed as to how best to approach this problem, much interest has turned to the identification of "high-risk pregnancies," with subsequent intensive care directed toward this group of patients (Nesbitt, 1966; Jacobson, 1964). Wider prenatal screening for subclinical entities such as urinary tract infection, diabetes, congenital heart disease, genital cancer, hypothyroidism, anemia, viral disease and genetic abnormalities has been added to previous routines for evaluation. Closer attention toward detection of venereal disease, with its recently increased prevalence, has been made mandatory. The role of drugs, genetics, habits and nutrition, with special attention to protein intake, has been stressed. Prenatal hospitalization for evaluation and control of special medical problems has assumed an increasingly important role. In addition to their basic medical value, such procedures have served to impress upon the patient the fact that the medical team is concerned about her pregnancy and maternal outcome, and have helped to draw her into a greater self-awareness and participation in solving her problems. Earlier consultation with the pediatric team, including prenatal consultations, and involvement of other appropriate specialists, have been found to have obvious advantages. In general, then, the increasing role of preventive medicine in obstetrics, with a concentrated interdisciplinary approach to the high-risk pregnancy group, has been the basis of the modern concept of prenatal care.

The obvious and logical next question, therefore, is whether or not the adolescent pregnancy is at high risk. In order to answer this question, it is appropriate to briefly review the relationships between sociological issues and the adequacy of medical care and pregnancy outcome. Because of the previously-mentioned desire to improve maternal and perinatal outcome, the past several years have seen the beginnings of attempts to explore sociological, as well as physiological, aspects of patient care (Osofsky, 1968, c, d). Numerous studies have related death rates to socioeconomic status. It has been conclusively shown that life expectancy at all levels can be correlated with social class. Tuberculosis, influenza, pneumonia, syphilis, and other infectious illnesses are all more common among the poor (Chase, 1965). Deaths from diabetes, cancer, nephritis, arteriosclerosis, and hypertension are also more common among the poor than they are among the affluent members of society (Chase, 1965; Shapiro, 1965). The statistics tend to dispel the misconception that some of these illnesses, such as hypertension, are diseases of middle-class executives. Whatever the complex reasons may be, the poor seem more prone to fatality.

Obstetrics has been no exception to the rule. Although death rates for mothers and infants have improved in all classes, the improvement in the more favored groups has been disproportionately higher than in the lower socioeconomic classes. The disparity is striking when the national rates for white patients are compared with those for blacks. The white maternal death rate (per 10,000 live births) decreased from 60 in 1930 to 2.1 in 1965; the black death rate decreased from 117 to 8.4 (Eastman, 1961; U.S. Dept. of Health, Education and Welfare, 1968). Correspondingly, the white fetal death rate (per 1,000 live births) fell from 35.1 in 1926 to 13.9 in 1965, while during the same period the nonwhite rate fell from 73 to 27.2 (Nesbitt, 1957; U.S. Dept. of Health, Education and Welfare, 1968). In addition to the absolute figures for mortality, poor patients tend to fare worse in general, with a higher incidence of morbidity in all measures, for both mothers and infants. Toxemia, anemia, excessive weight gain, and prematurity, for example, all have higher incidences among poor patients (Chase, 1965; Nesbit, 1957). The infants born to poor mothers have a higher incidence of morbidity in all parameters

TABLE IV

FETAL, NEONATAL AND PERINATAL DEATH RATES BY COLOR
AND YEAR IN THE UNITED STATES

Year	Fetal Deaths*		Neonatal Deaths*		Perinatal Deaths*	
	White	Nonwhite	White	Nonwhite	White	Nonwhite
1940	NA	NA	27.2	39.7	NA+	NA+
1945	21.4	42.0	23.3	32.0	54.7	74.0
1950	17.1	32.5	19.4	27.5	36.5	60.0
1955	15.2	28.4	17.7	27.2	32.9	45.6
1960	14.1	26.8	17.2	26.9	31.3	53.7
1965	13.9	27.2	16.1	25.4	30.0	52.6

* Deaths per 1,000 live births
  Abstracted from Department of Health, Education and Welfare Vital Statistics
Reports

studied; and, perhaps related to less adequate nutrition of the mothers, signs of malnutrition in the infants are more commonly found at birth (Donabedian, 1965; Drillien, 1964; North, 1966).

As a result of the factors which have been previously mentioned, it would be expected that pregnant teen-agers would fall into this sociologically high-risk population, even if patient age were not of importance itself in prognosticating pregnancy outcome. Because of the many factors, such as abortion, which tend to exclude middle and upper socioeconomic girls from the overall figures concerning teen-age pregnancy, the bulk of teen-age pregnancies, especially those within the unmarried category, occur in members of the lower socioeconomic class. Further, as already stated, these figures indicate that, at least among the unwed groups, 60 percent are nonwhite and only 40 percent are white. Because of these facts, the unwed pregnant teen-ager is doubly jeopardized medically. By being a member of a lower socioeconomic class, her incidence of all pregnancy complications and perinatal wastage is significantly increased. Further, if she is in addition nonwhite, her chances are worse again. These complications do not even take into account possible adverse affects related to the youth of the patients. In order to better understand the influences of the combined factors of age, illegitimacy, lower socioeconomic class, and ethnic background, it would seem worthwhile to first look at medical results of teen-age pregnancies in the United States.

A REVIEW OF TEEN-AGE PREGNANCY RESULTS

With few exceptions, studies do indeed support the notion that adolescent pregnant females are at high risk medically. One of the few exceptions is a report from England, by Stearn (1963). He carefully followed 30 unwed primiparas under the age of 16 and found that, in general, the mothers did well. Of interest, though, in spite of the overall favorable outcome, even in his group there was increased incidence of excessive weight gain, hypertension, and toxemia. Most American authors have reported considerably more grim findings than those of Stearn. The reader is referred to the studies of Claman (1964), Aznar (1961), Mussio (1962), Polliakoff (1958), and Semmens (1965). Each of these authors has reviewed his work with pregnant teenagers and, on the whole, multiple problems such as an increased incidence of prematurity, disproportion, excessive weight gain, hypertension, and especially toxemia, have been noted.

Four studies warrant special consideration because they demonstrate some of the problems which are faced because of the complex interweaving of illegitimacy, socioeconomic background, ethnic origin, and age. The first, reported by Pakter (1961b) has dealt primarily with the issue of illegitimacy. In this study, an analysis was made of live birth and infant death certificates in New York City for the year 1955 through 1959. Within the large group, almost all complications of pregnancy occurred more frequently among the unmarried than among the married women. The incidence of both toxemia and hypertension were 50 percent greater among the unmarried groups. The puerperal maternal death rate was approximately four times as great for the unmarried (21.3 per 10,000 live births) as for the married (5.0 per 10,000 live births). Some of this impressively major differential in maternal death rate can be accounted for by the inclusion of deaths secondary to illegal abortions within the overall figures. However, even after excluding abortions, the death rate was almost twice as great for the unmarried mothers than it was for those who were married. Both prematurity and perinatal mortality rates were considerably higher among infants born out of wedlock than among infants delivered to married mothers. The significance of this increased incidence of prematurity and perinatal mortality will be more fully discussed in a subsequent section.

In her report, Pakter has also demonstrated that a considerable proportion of the differences between married and unmarried groups are related to socioeconomic background and to ethnic derivation. Nonwhites in general had markedly greater incidences of all complications reported than did white women of similar marital status. However, within ethnic and economic subgroups, the reported complications were still considerably more common for the unmarried mothers and their offspring than they were for the married.

TABLE V

NEONATAL DEATH RATES BY RACE AND AGE OF MOTHER
BALTIMORE RESIDENTS, 1961

	Neonatal Death Rates		
Age of Mother	White	Nonwhite	Total
16 years and under	23.0	42.8	35.8
17—19	20.3	33.8	27.5
20 and over	16.9	27.4	21.7
Total	17.4	27.4	21.7

From Stine (1964)

The second study to be cited is by Stine (1964). In his report, he reviewed records for Baltimore residents during 1961, and has compared neonatal and prematurity rates on the basis of age and race of mothers. His figures reveal marked differences on the basis of both parameters. The overall racial breakdown demonstrates an incidence of a prematurity of 7.6 percent among the white and 14.2 percent among the nonwhite mothers, and a neonatal death rate of 17.4 per 1,000 live births among the white and 29.5 per 1,000 live births among the nonwhite mothers.

The breakdown, on the basis of age, reveals differences in the anticipated direction. The overall rate of prematurity for all groups studied was 10.8 percent. For the two younger groups it was appreciably higher: 17 to 19 year old mothers experienced a prematurity rate of 13.9 percent; mothers under 17 experienced a rate of 18.1 percent. For all groups, regardless of age, the neonatal mortality rate was 23.2 per 1,000 live births. For infants delivered to mothers aged 17 through 19, the figure was 27.5 per 1,000 live births; for infants of mothers under 17 the figure reached 35.8 per 1,000 live births.

When one combines the two parameters of age and race, as would so often be the case with teen-age mothers, the figures become even more striking. Among white mothers, age 17 through 19, the incidence of prematurity was 8.6 percent; among nonwhite mothers the incidence was 17.3 percent. Among white mothers under 17, the incidence of prematurity was 11.1 percent; among nonwhite mothers it was 20.3 percent.

The figures reported do not have an additional breakdown upon the basis of maternal economic status. If such were available, it might be anticipated that these results would also be striking. However, Stine's data clearly indicates that age and racial factors, separately and together, serve to influence the incidences of both prematurity and neonatal mortality.

Battaglia (1963), in another study, has reviewed all deliveries at the Johns Hopkins Hospital during the years 1939 through 1960, and has broken down the statistics by maternal age at the time of delivery. Similarly, Hassan (1964), has reviewed the pregnancies of 159 young primiparas in Chicago, and has compared their course to older primiparas and to patients in general, regardless of parity. Both authors have demonstrated a markedly increased incidence of excessive weight gain, toxemia, prolonged labor, cervical laceration, Cesarean section, prematurity, and perinatal mortality.

As one looks at the four reports which have been specifically cited, one finds consistent and dramatic results. Maternal youthful age, by itself, does appear to be related to a higher incidence of pregnancy complications and maternal and fetal wastage. When one adds on the compounding factors of poverty, illegitimacy, and non-white background, one is indeed dealing with a

TABLE VI
PREMATURITY RATES BY AGE OF MOTHER
BALTIMORE STUDY

Age of Mother	Percent Premature Deliveries
Less than 15 years (1951—1960)	23.4
15—19 years (1951—1960)	18.3
All ages (1960)	16.3

Abstracted from Battaglia (1963)

group of pregnancies at extremely high risk from the obstetrician's point of view.

From a medical point of view, it must be emphasized that not only are adolescent mothers at high risk, but it appears that their infants are similarly in jeopardy. As has been pointed out, there is a much higher incidence of prematurity in pregnancies occurring in the teen-age population. This prematurity is of marked significance. On one hand, it undoubtedly relates to the high incidence of perinatal wastage (which has already been cited) among the delivered infants. Pakter (1961b), for example, in her series, reports an infant mortality rate of 195.0 per 1,000 live births among out-of-wedlock prematures as compared with a rate of 17.1 per 1,000 live births among out-of-wedlock infants delivered at term. It is worth noting that prematurity, in addition to contributing to infant wastage, has other, and perhaps equally ominous, medical implications.

Knoblock and Pasamanick (Knoblock, 1962, 1966; Pasamanick, 1959, 1966), in the United States, and Drillien (1959, 1964), in Scotland, have in very extensive studies each found a markedly increased incidence of both mental subnormality and neurological deficit in surviving premature infants. When birth weight is 3 pounds or less, the incidence of major neurological deficit and mental subnormality requiring special schooling or institutionalization may run as high as 20 percent.

The more recent study by Drillien (1964) has further demonstrated the important finding that by age five most premature infants in middle and upper socioeconomic classes have caught up with their peers. Where social developmental conditions are not as favorable, the incidence of persistent problems, if anything, tends to increase. Such conditions include: deprived socioeconomic environment, other small offspring in the family, overcrowding of the home, poor maternal and/or paternal stimulation, and illegitimacy. Obviously, all of the above-mentioned complicating factors are frequent complications of adolescent pregnancies.

In addition to the infant morbidity and mortality problems which are related to prematurity, there appear to be further difficulties which are associated with the out-of-wedlock condition itself and which are compounded by poverty and ethnic background. Pakter (1961b), for example, has correlated infant death rates due to respiratory infections and accidents to these conditions. She has found that the death rate due to these causes is more than twice as common among infants born out of wedlock than among infants delivered to married mothers. Again, poverty and ethnic background are important contributors to these figures. But, illegitimacy, itself, seems to play a distinct role.

Further, Pasamanick (1966) and Knobloch (1966) have correlated the development of subsequent mental subnormality and multiple neurological difficulties with general pregnancy complications, as well as prematurity. All of the studied mental and neurological difficulties showed a higher incidence when general pregnancy complications existed. Pasamanick and Knobloch have pointed out that these conditions occur more commonly among the poor, the nonwhite, the unwed, and especially among teen-age mothers. On the basis of their findings, Pasamanick and Knobloch have singled out pregnancies in low socioeconomic groups as being of high risk as far as the developmental prognosis of the infant is concerned, and further singled out infants of teen-age mothers as being in greatest jeopardy of all infants studied.

COMPOUNDING FACTORS WHICH INFLUENCE MEDICAL PROGNOSIS

The question can be raised as to why pregnant teen-age mothers and their infants are at such high risk medically. Perhaps, in part, the difficulties are related to the state of adolescence itself. Although the very ability to conceive in itself suggests a considerable degree of physiologic maturation, certainly the adolescent is in a state of flux physiologically and metabolically. Many of the organ systems, such as the thyroid gland and the pancreas, are already under stress in adolescence; the effects of the additional stress of pregnancy are unknown. The bony pelvis is relatively mature radiologically, but the high incidence of disproportion suggests that full growth has not been completed. Similarly, the high incidence of prematurity and other pregnancy complications suggests that the uterus itself, together with its interrelationships with other organs, may not be functioning in precisely the same manner in the early and midteens as would be true at a slightly later stage of life. Further, adolescence is known to be a stage of life which is compounded by poor nutritional habits. In pregnancy, where diet is of such major importance, these poor habits assume even greater significance.

In addition, since many of the early- and mid-teen-age pregnancies occur out of wedlock, and since out-of-wedlock pregnancy connotes social unacceptability, many patients have numerous social, emotional, and economic problems, all of which can be expected to delay the patient's seeking and accepting medical care. Further, since many of the patients who neither illegally abort themselves nor enter a nursing home are poor and/or nonwhite, there is the very real question of the adequacy of the metabolic and nutritional background prior to the pregnancy. In many, there is obviously a dietary deficiency of long standing (Birch, 1967; Dibble, 1965; Mayer, 1965). The parameters which lead to nutritional inadequacy have far-reaching implications. Studies of both animals and humans suggest that inadequate maternal nutrition contributes to infants of smaller birth weight, with more neonatal complications, and difficulty with developmental problems at a later date (Crovito, 1966; Crowley, 1959; Donabedian, 1965; North, 1966; Smith, 1964; Waranky, 1944).

Faced with this complex picture of the interaction between the physiologic difficulties of adolescence itself, and those secondary to ethnic and socioeconomic backgrounds of pregnant adolescents, it is logical to assume that the quality and intensity of medical care is of considerable importance in determining the prognosis of the pregnancy. It becomes particularly ominous to look at the figures for antenatal care among pregnant teen-agers. Pakter (1961a), in her review of out-of-wedlock pregnancies in New York City, has demonstrated that, whereas 45.7 percent of all married women receive antenatal care by the end of the first trimester of pregnancy, only 6.6 percent of out-of-wedlock mothers receive such care. The figures at the end of the sixth month of pregnancy are just as striking: 87.2 percent of married women have received care by this stage of pregnancy, whereas fewer than 50 percent of women pregnant out of wedlock have received any care. Among whites, the figures are somewhat different, although in the same direction, as they are among nonwhites: 87.2 percent of married white women have received some care by the end of six months of pregnancy, as compared to 61.7 percent of married nonwhites. Among married women, the figures are slightly worse for the whites, with 36.7 percent of white and 42.9 percent of nonwhite women having received care during the first six months of pregnancy. Of some note, 14.7 percent of women pregnant out of wedlock have received no prenatal care, as opposed to 4 percent of married women. The infant death rate for out-of-wedlock infants whose mothers have received no prenatal care is 116.6 per 1,000 live births as opposed to 32.2 per 1,000 live births for out-of-wedlock infants whose mothers have received some care.

The reasons for the inadequacy of prenatal care are related to several factors. One of the most important factors is that of ethnic background and socioeconomic class. As has been mentioned, a high percentage of pregnant adolescents who carry their pregnancies to term are nonwhite and poor. Even when adolescence is excluded, various authors have demonstrated health care differences on the basis of socioeconomic class and have attempted to explore the etiology of these differences.

Koos (1954), in a study of small community living, has demonstrated that socioeconomic class appears to affect patient attitudes toward medical symptoms. The higher the patient's class, the more likely is he to consult a physician for a specific symptom. The lowest socioeconomic class appears to show a marked indifference to symptoms. Especially when symptoms neither interfere with work nor cause disabling pain, poor patients are much less likely than are the more affluent to consider themselves able to consult a physician.

Another patient-oriented factor which may interfere with the effectiveness of medical care received is described in a review by Simmons (1957), who points out that public health precepts are based upon middle-class norms, and that lower-class norms may interfere with effective functioning of public health activity. Middle-class norms place a high value on ability to defer gratifications in the interest of long-range goals. Simmons states that lower-class patients may not have the readiness to sacrifice the present for possible gains in the future. This priority for immediate rewards has important implications in obstetrics, in which so much of the care is of a preventative nature, and in which the patient is asked to defer gratification (for example, in quantitative and qualitative eating habits) for a prolonged time in order to achieve better health for both the mother and the offspring.

Simmons further discusses the middle-class norm of a strong sense of individual responsibility. This contrasts with the lower socioeconomic class in which the kin group is seen as being partially responsible for the patient's well-being.

In several articles, the question of the individual's definition of health and illness is raised. Koos demonstrates the problem in relation to physician consultation by patients for specific symptoms. Simmons (1957), Wellin (1958), and Paul (1963) all refer to difficulties in eradicating disease because of folk medicine concepts which are different from modern scientific medical concepts. A disease such as typhus has posed problems for a public health team entering a community, because of the inhabitants' inability to believe that a relatively nonobtrusive insect can be related to major physical symptoms. This difficulty is further compounded when other insects or hazards exist in the environment which produce more pain or discomfort to the patient.

Kutner (1961) points out that lack of knowledge of the importance of symptoms results in a marked delay for the poor in seeking medical care. In his study, the patients all had cancer; among the poor the disease was often more widespread at the time of the initial visit because of the patient's lack of awareness of the significance of the symptoms. (It should be mentioned that Kutner's results do not take into account the possibility that middle-class patients have frequent periodic prophylactic check-ups and that these checkups may further contribute to earlier diagnosis of significant disease among the more affluent. This does not, however, negate Kutner's conclusions.)

Obviously, the implication of such findings is of major importance to a field such as obstetrics. With patient difficulty both in accepting the need to defer gratifications, and in interpreting the importance of non-disabling conditions such as weight gain, edema, albuminuria, and hypertension, one barrier to receiving effective and comprehensive care is obvious. It is worth mentioning, that though these findings may generally be true, there are individual differences within the broad group which compromises the lower socioeconomic class. Mechanic (1960) has found considerable individual variation due to background, education, and familial individual attitudes. In general, though, class-related differences appear to be consistent.

Another obvious and major factor which is related to the patient's achieving appropriate care is that of quality of care offered. In spite of changing social legislation, the majority of poor patients receive care in a clinic atmosphere. Visits may require a several hour wait in an impersonal waiting room. Often when the doctor is seen, he has but a few minutes to offer the patient. Further, the patient commonly sees a different doctor at each visit, and as a result there are difficulties in establishing the traditional doctor-patient relationship, with which the middle and upper classes are familiar. Bernstein (1963), has pointed out that the impersonal atmosphere of clinics and the long waiting times which they foster are responsible for many patient cancellations and a general disinterest in keeping appointments.

The issue of the doctor-patient relationship may, however, have even further implications than those suggested by the clinic atmosphere. Parsons (1963), has discussed the traditional American concept of the warm and individual doctor-patient relationship. The patient under this system is expected to desire to get well and to cooperate fully with the physician. The physician is expected to be completely devoted to the welfare of his patient, and to come to terms with him as an individual. He is expected to emphasize patient welfare at all times. Although the clinic atmosphere might be expected to interfere with the establishment of individual deep relationships, by itself it would not necessarily destroy the image of the doctor as being a dedicated individual who has as his sole interest the desire to help the patient get well.

Of interest, therefore, is Koos' (1954) observation that low status persons feel that physicians don't want them as patients. Such an accusation, if true, would obviously be in conflict with the anticipated doctor-patient relationship described by Parsons.

That the low status patient may be differently perceived by physicians, and may indeed be given less adequate care is borne out by the studies done by Redlich (1955), Myers (1954), and Osofsky (1968c, d). The first two of these studies deal with patients in a psychiatric clinic. Both studies indicate that even when economic background is similar, patients receive differential treatment related to their degree of *social desirability*. The patients who least successfully meet the personnel's definition of a good patient have considerably longer waiting times prior to being accepted for treatment, and, in addition, receive less intensive treatment. The third study suggests that, as might be expected, obstetrical patients undergo a similar experience. Resident and practicing physician comments indicate a differential in both perception and treatment of poor patients, especially those of low *social desirability*. For example, the *poor* graduate student's wife is more likely to receive optimal care than is the *poor* laborer's wife, especially if the latter does not dress neatly or otherwise conform to middle-class standards. Simmons (1957), describing programs for underdeveloped countries, makes similar findings:

> It appears that the degree to which the qualities ideally defined as essential to the therapeutic relationship, namely mutual trust, respect and cooperation, will be present in a given professional patient relationship varies with the amount of social distance. Conversely, the greater the social distance, the less likely that the participants will perceive each other in terms of ideal type role of professional

and patient and the more likely that they will perceive each other in terms of their social class status in the larger society.

Thus, specific problems in obtaining appropriate medical care, related to the social class of the patients, are present. The problems are partially those of the patients. Differences in motivation, perception of symptoms, perceptions of need for prophylactic medical care, and, perhaps, under some circumstances a lesser willingness to assume individual responsibility, are all factors contributing to a lower quality of medical care. These patient factors are related to individual norms and lack of medical sophistication.

A second set of factors are those related to the type of care received—the impersonal clinic with its long waits and constantly changing physicians.

But, it must be emphasized that still a third class of factors exists. It does seem that the medical team differentially perceives and treats lower socioeconomic class patients. Physicians and other medical personnel seem to prefer patients from middle and upper socioeconomic classes. The quality of care offered to poorer patients by necessity suffers. Therefore, as has been stated, a complex interweaving of factors—patient, facility, and medical team—intertwine in a manner which contributes to the higher morbidity and mortality existing for lower socioeconomic patients.

In addition to racial and economic factors, further difficulties exist related to the status of adolescence itself. Even in the nonpregnant state, the adolescent presents a perplexing medical problem. On one hand, adolescents feel uncomfortable in the usual pediatric office, surrounded by infants and young children; at the same time, they may feel just as uncomfortable in the waiting room of the physician whose practice is primarily devoted to adults, with a large component of middle-aged and elderly patients filling the waiting room. Thus, adolescence remains the era of life in which medical care is least often sought out; as a result, throughout the country there exists a supervision gap in adolescent medicine.

Compounding this problem are the specific issues related to those individuals who represent the pregnant teen-agers. As has been pointed out, teen-age pregnancy may occur in any socioeconomic class and under any circumstance. However, when one eliminates some of the more favored groups, namely the older married teen-agers, those who undergo abortion, and those with enough ability and financial independence to stay in a maternity home, one is left with a biased population. The chapter on education will cover in greater depth the problems such girls have with school achievement, truancy, and even delinquency. A considerable percentage have had difficulty in the past in relating to authority figures, such as welfare workers, who may have behaved in a punitive manner. At least, the girls would typically be on guard, since information contained in workers' reports could result in the loss of welfare assistance. It is neither unlikely nor suprising that difficulties continue in relationships between medical authorities and patients during teen-age pregnancies.

A further concept which must be considered is the attitude of the pregnant teen-ager toward herself. A notion has developed which defines pregnant teen-agers, especially those from lower socioeconomic and nonwhite groups, as being nonchalant about being pregnant out of wedlock. The nonwhite girl, together with her family, is supposed to be unconcerned, or even proud, about the prospect of being pregnant and having a baby to love. Illegitimacy, according to this view, is no shame (Childers, 1936). At this time it would be appropriate to mention that such interpretations are, to a great extent, misconceptions. There is little evidence to suggest that, at the present time, in this country, pregnant unwed teen-agers, regardless of race and socioeconomic class, do not feel some degree of shame of social stigma (Bernard, 1966; Hertz, 1944; Himes, 1964; Osili, 1957).

Commonly there are family pressures of disappointment. Almost always there are partly hidden and even openly-directed punitive actions from other authority figures within the community. The girl is forced to leave school. Peers of both sexes may behave differently and somewhat judgmentally. Teachers and principals may exhibit a critical and punitive air. Regardless of whether society's standards are the best, the girl is aware that she has deviated from them, and that, in some ways, she is an outcast. If one adds on to these feelings other adolescent anxieties and rebellious traits, and when one compounds the issue further including the ambivalent feelings of low socioeconomic patients to physicians and medical personnel, the stage is set for increased difficulties in accepting medical care. The patients are ashamed, and afraid of what the feelings of the medical team to them will be. In the past their experience has often been that of long waits, impersonal physicians, and, in short, no medical person to whom they could positively relate.

Adding to these problems may be the actual attitudes of the medical teams. If we remember that physicians and nurses react as adults, who are members of their own social class, in addition to reacting appropriately as professionals, we are faced with the realization that medical personnel may add to the pregnant teen-agers' problems.

Medical personnel may have trouble dealing with poor and nonwhite patients; there may be further difficulties related to dealing with teen-agers in general. Whatever attitudes exist toward teen-agers, per se, will be magnified and distorted when the medical condition is that of unwed pregnancy. Unwed pregnancy in the teen-ager stirs up anxieties about sexuality, promiscuity, and intercourse among the young, as well as moral feelings about illegitimacy. It is possible, without conscious awareness, for the medical personnel to behave judgmentally and punitively toward the pregnant teen-ager.

One example which makes such a suggestion plausible is the utilization of the term *recidivism* to refer to repeated unwed pregnancy. This term, which is used so commonly, is defined by the dictionary as "the repeating of a crime even after the individual has received adequate punishment for the crime." Whether or not repeat teen-age pregnancy is inappropriate, obviously few physicians and nurses would consciously describe it as a crime. Yet, just as the term which is used to define the condition has a criminal connotation, it would be surprising if the medical team did not often inadvertently react with anxiety and even disapproval to the condition of unmarried teen-age pregnancy. Such reactions serve to reinforce teen-agers' existing anxiety, tend to make it more difficult for them to relate to

medical personnel, and thus further lessen the chances for adequate medical care.

Thus we see evolving a complex set of intertwining conditions,
all of which act to interfere with pregnant teen-agers receiving
adequate medical care. There are barriers on the basis of socioeconomic class, race, and age. There are barriers which emanate
from the patient and her family; there are additional barriers,
not only from society, but from the medical team in particular.
Obviously all of these barriers—in addition to any specific
physiological, metabolic, and nutritional problems of teen-
agers—contribute to the pregnant teen-agers' and the unborn
infants' being at risk. Just as obviously, major efforts need to be
made if any diminution of this risk is to be accomplished.

SOME SOLUTIONS TO MINIMIZE MEDICAL RISK

Of some note, in light of the abundant data which has demonstrated both the difficulty and unfavorable prognosis for pregnant teen-agers and their infants, are the early results of the
Y-MED program (Braen, 1968; Osofsky, 1967a; 1968a, b), which
is introduced in the preface.

Y-MED has been available to all girls desirous of its services.
However, because it has operated in some ways as a day care
center within the community, it has attracted primarily those
girls who are not concealing their pregnancies. As a result, the
overwhelming majority of the girls have come from lower socioeconomic areas of the community; of the first 225 girls entering
the program, 85 percent have received some welfare assistance
and 70 percent have been nonwhite. (Of some interest, with
greater community acceptance of the program, there has been
a gradual shift in the racial background of the girls within the
program. During the first year, 90 percent of the girls were
nonwhite; during the second year, 70 percent were nonwhite;
during the third year, approximately 60 percent were nonwhite.)

Knowing that adolescent pregnancies are medically at high
risk because of multiple reasons, the medical staff has set up a
unique program at Y-MED. The overall concept of the program

has been geared to provide an extremely broad-based service with a high degree of both intensity and personal attention. An attempt has been made to give girls care from the earliest possible point in pregnancy; this care has been continued throughout the pregnancy, labor, delivery, and first year postpartum. In addition, a nursery has been provided with the three-fold goal of giving infant care in order that the mothers may return to school, of creating good standards of infant medical care and stimulation during the first year of life, and of creating an atmosphere which can hopefully allow the mothers to learn good techniques of child care.

From the start, the traditional clinic concept has been abandoned. The medical program has operated within the framework of a medical center teaching program, but the girls have been treated as private patients. This has been done both in an attempt to provide more effective medical care and to allow the patients to establish meaningful relationships with physicians—perhaps the first meaningful patient-physician relationships in their lives. Senior residents and full-time faculty have served as permanent physicians in a group practice arrangement. These physicians meet the girls at the initial visit, and then follow them throughout the pregnancy, labor, delivery and the postpartal period. The girls have specific appointments to see their doctors, with no long waits in an impersonal room. If an emergency develops, a patient can call her physician through a 24-hour answering service. When labor begins, again the individual relationship prevails. The girl's doctor is called; he comes to the hospital and follows the girl as any other private patient would be followed.

Pediatric care has been arranged in a similar manner. Instructors in pediatrics have served as the program pediatricians. During the course of the pregnancy, each girl meets individually with them to discuss future pediatric needs. If the labor or delivery is complicated, a pediatrician is in attendance at the hospital along with the obstetrician. After delivery, the same physicians care for the infants in the hospital, visiting the mothers and informing them of progress. When the children return home and to the day nursery, the pediatrician carefully supervises their care.

In addition to formal medical care, the physicians, nurses, and other medical personnel conduct classes three times weekly for the girls. Within these classes, the girls are taught basic facts about themselves and their infants, including data on their bodies, pregnancy, delivery, infant care, and psychological development.

A minimum of three weekly general staff conferences are held. All members of the program meet to discuss general issues and specific patient problems at these meetings. At these sessions long-range goals for the girls are formulated. In all matters, as has been mentioned, the program is "girl-oriented." The staff attempts to work for the girls' needs and not their own. Whatever is best for each individual girl is always the major consideration.

As has been mentioned, the enrollment of the girls within the program has indicated a traditionally high-risk population. Three percent of the girls have been twelve or thirteen; 19 percent fourteen to fifteen; 56 percent sixteen to seventeen; 20 percent eighteen to nineteen; and 2 percent have been twenty years of age.

To date, 175 girls have fully participated in the medical program (an additional 50 had participated in limited educational and social service aspects of the program before the medical program was fully operational). Of the girls in the medical program, 100 have now delivered a total of 102 infants (two sets of twins). As hoped for, the majority of the girls have been seen early in the course of pregnancy. Forty-seven percent have received medical care by the twentieth week of pregnancy, and only 8 percent have had no care prior to the last ten weeks of pregnancy. The average number of prenatal visits has been thirteen per girl. The hoped for relationships between patients and doctors have often developed.

In spite of the intensive medical care, a greater number of complications have been observed than could be expected in a routine population. Twenty-four percent of the girls have required antenatal hospitalization because of complications of pregnancy. Incipient or early toxemia, excessive weight gain, and anemia have been frequent problems. Although complications have occurred somewhat more frequently than would be anticipated from a population at large, they have been considerably less common than might have been anticipated on the basis of the reports already cited concerning similar populations. Prematurity by weight has complicated 14.7 percent of the pregnancies; when non-premature twins and small-for-dates infants are excluded, the rate falls to 6.9 percent. Either figure is considerably lower than those previously cited for similar groups.

TABLE VII

Y-MED (YOUNG MOTHERS EDUCATIONAL DEVELOPMENT) PROGRAM
MEDICAL RESULTS FOR FIRST 100 DELIVERIES

Number of Infants Delivered	102 (2 sets of twins)
Number of Patients With Hemoglobin Below 12	64
Number of Patients With Hemoglobin Below 10	14
Number of Patients With Insipient or Mild Toxemia	11
Number of Diagnosed Urinary Tract Infections	5
Number of Antenatal Hospitalizations Excluding False Labor	34
Number of Cesarean Sections	7
Number of Prematures (Less Than 2500 Grams)	15
Number of Prematures by Weight and Dates (excluding twins and small-for-dates infants)	8
Incidence of Perinatal Mortality	0

Further, in spite of frequent minor complications, only one major complication has been reported in the entire series, a girl who had postpartal subinvolution requiring nine units of blood. In addition, to the time of writing of this manuscript, there has not been a single perinatal mortality in the program. Obviously, this finding of absent perinatal mortality will not last forever. In any normal population, there is bound to be a low incidence of perinatal mortality if enough deliveries are performed. However, the absence of perinatal mortality to the present time, together with the diminution of other problems, is most exciting since obviously a higher percentage of complications could be anticipated within this population. Thus, obstetrically, it would appear that progress is being made.

Pediatrically, it is still too early to give detailed results. Many of the infants are still very young. At the present time a careful maturational and developmental assessment is being performed upon all of the infants. The results should be available in the not-too-distant future. A broad statement can be made, however, at the present time. The babies appear to be responding well to the pediatric care; the mothers appear to be carefully following the pediatrician's advice. The infants are thriving and seem to be developing normally. At the present time, there is only one case of even suspected retardation in the entire group.

The results which have been cited are not meant to indicate that programs such as Y-MED are the only or even the best answer to the medical problems of pregnant teen-agers. The results do indicate, however, that an intensive, sensitive, and respectful effort can be successful in ameliorating many of the medical problems experienced by both groups of extremely high-risk patients—the pregnant teen-agers and their infants.

Two other programs, both of which have been designed to provide intensive and meaningful medical experience, have been reporting similarly good obstetrical results. These are at Yale Medical Center in New Haven, Connecticut, and at Mt. Sinai Hospital in New York City. Each program has been in existence for a short period, and each is already reporting figures indicating relatively low rates of complications, a diminished incidence of prematurity, and absent perinatal mortality (Sarrel, 1967, personal communication). Again, it is emphasized that the problems related to age, illegitimacy, poverty, and ethnic background are of major importance. No program can serve as a panacea for these problems. No program can eliminate all of the difficulties which are related to these problems. No program can negate the data which demonstrate the extreme risk which these individuals present for themselves and their infants. However, the early data which each of these unusual programs presents demonstrates that meaningful efforts can result in a successful lessening of problems.

Other efforts obviously need to be made to combat the fundamental medical problems which are related to poverty. Educational efforts need to be intensified both for patients and for the medical personnel who deal with these patients. More effort needs to be made to reach those who are classified as *"unreach-*

able." But at the same time, similar efforts are necessary to instruct those who will provide services to those-so-called *unreachables*.

In addition to the metabolic, physiologic, and nutritional difficulties which need to be corrected, the bigotry which exists both on the part of patients and medical personnel needs to be eradicated before the problems of these and other high-risk individuals can be solved. Some limited steps have been made. Others of a more fundamental nature still remain to be taken.

III

THE SOCIAL SERVICE PROBLEM

In the preceding section on medical problems of the pregnant teen-ager, one of the concepts that emerged was that of high-risk pregnancy. We saw that those girls who are prognostically at highest risk medically—because of age, race, and socioeconomic class—are likely to receive the poorest medical attention. (Of course they may be of medical high risk to start with because of both poor nutritional background and less than optimal prior medical care.)

The bleak picture is similar in the area of social service. Those persons in the society who need social service most—get it least.

Are the pregnant teen-agers at high risk from a social service point of view? A wide array of authors have approached this question; they seem to conclude *yes*.

A RESEARCH REVIEW

To some extent, as Vincent (1961) has pointed out, there is a marked selectivity in certain studies which relate to the decade in which the investigations were carried out. Prior to 1930, emphasis was placed upon immorality, bad companions, and mental deficiency. Studies of that era were descriptive; subjects were often mothers in rescue homes and other types of charity institutions. As might be expected from such studies, the conclusions, on the whole, confirmed the hypotheses concerning the etiology of illegitimacy. (Bingham, 1923; Guiford, 1922; Lowe, 1927; McClure, 1931; Mangold, 1921; Schumacher, 1927).

During the 1930's, environmental contributions to behavior assumed more importance in thinking and research activity. Studies of this decade frequently dealt with the relationships between broken homes, poverty, and unfavorable conditions, and subsequent illegitimacy. Of some note, these studies often relied upon court files, police records, welfare agency information, and data from homes for *wayward girls*. As one looks at the populations which were used in these studies, it is not at all surprising that again the hypotheses of the authors concerning the etiology of illegitimacy were confirmed. (Nottingham, 1937; Puttey, 1937; Reed, 1934).

In the late 1930's and early 1940's, studies approached the problem of illegitimacy from the perspective of cultural backgrounds which might be accepting, and even encouraging, of illegitimacy. Such studies frequently relied upon the anthropological techniques of focusing on communities, national regions, and even island cultures. These studies pointed out that the southern slave system had fostered a pattern of living within which middle-class family structures were relatively nonexistent. One stable male was seldom present in this situation, and illegitimacy was fostered, and in some areas, even encouraged by the plantation owners for economic and social reasons. On the basis of such background data, it was claimed that blacks, having recently been descended from this slave culture, were more accepting and permissive of the status of illegitimacy (Billingsley, 1966; Frazier, 1937; Hertz, 1944; Jenkins, 1958; Johnson, 1946; Kansanin, 1941; Knapp, 1944; Myrdal, 1944; Powdermaker, 1939). Studies done in Caribbean communities emerged with similar conclusions. There were areas in the Caribbean Islands where the rate of illegitimacy was relatively high, and in those areas, illegitimacy was condoned. The researchers, therefore, hypothesized that the condoning of illegitimacy within some Caribbean island communities could be related to the relatively high incidence of illegitimacy which occurs among Puerto Ricans in the United States (Goode, 1960; Herskovits, 1947; Smith, 1956; Rodman, 1963). Thus, at least for some authors, the association became a simple one. Permissive cultures, which were often matriarchal and not far removed from slavery, and which further did not condemn illegitimacy, etiologically resulted in high rates of illegitimacy among their members, not only in times gone by but even with present day Negroes and Puerto Ricans.

During the later 1940's and 1950's, psychological and psychiatric studies became more popular in general; these studies gained a special prominence in relationship to the etiology of illegitimacy. Frequently, authors attempted to define teen-age, out-of-wedlock pregnancy as being a symptomatic and purposeful attempt by the individual girl to solve an unresolved conflict. It was claimed that out-of-wedlock pregnancy was a symptom of underlying emotional difficulty. The hypothesis was presented that the teen-ager, in attempting to solve subconscious conflicts, acted out and became pregnant. It was stated that although the girl did not plan consciously to bear an out-of-wedlock child, she behaved in a manner which almost inevitably resulted in the unwanted pregnancy. She and her sexual partner might fail to utilize contraception during intercourse. Yet the girl subsequently claimed amazement and shock about the resulting pregnancy. Poor relationships with parents, including dominant mothers, passive mothers, aggressive fathers, passive fathers, or absent parents, were all presented as possible causes for the girl's acting out behavior. These studies were often done in maternity homes, welfare agencies, and outpatient clinics, where psychiatric social workers, clinical psychologists, and psychiatrists talked to individual clients. Often the clients were undergoing therapy, and their case histories were shared. Again, as would be expected from studies involving individuals under therapy, therapeutically-oriented researchers, and the types of facilities utilized, the data confirmed the hypotheses which had initially been offered (Block, 1945; Bonan, 1963; Cattell, 1954; Clothier, 1943; Deutsch, 1945; Donnell, 1952; Hutchinson, 1949; Kasanin, 1941; Lehfeldt, 1959; May, 1950; Young, 1945).

The middle and late 1950's and early 1960's have been marked by a renewed interest in the concept of the "society-as-patient." Such studies have focused upon difficulties which are inherently present in all classes. They have dealt with the morality or lack of morality which exists in present day society. Stress has been placed upon the growing inability of individuals to identify with

society at large during a time of rapid industrialization, automation, and the subsequent shrinking of the world. The concept
of anomie, especially among the lower classes, has been stressed;
social maladjustment within all groups, regardless of socioeconomic breakdown, has also been given emphasis. These studies
have come from physicians in private practice, workers in community agencies, and sociologists. Often the studies have mini-
mized class differences. There has been a tendency to cite the
similarities which exist between unwed mothers, and females
within the general population who are not pregnant out of wedlock (Anderson, 1957; Bernstein, 1960; Edlin, 1954; Gebhard,
1958; Pearson, 1956; Schauffler, 1955; Schmideberg, 1951; Vincent, 1961; Young, 1954).

This breakdown of research somewhat simplifies the approaches used in data collection. Obviously, there has been considerable overlap of work done at various times. This does not
negate the validity of noting the tendency for trends to occur,
regarding both popular hypotheses and types of research.

By categorizing the studies in this manner, I am not attempting to discredit their worth. Many have importance at the present
time. However, the approaches taken must result in questions
concerning validity. These questions are not specific to the
studies cited, but in general plague researchers interested in
obtaining data of sociological relevancy.

VALIDITY AND BIAS

Social science research suffers in general from a confusion
between internal and external validity (Campbell, 1957, 1963).
Whereas an experiment may be carefully done and produce in-
ternally valid conclusions, one should be careful when generalizing from the conclusions to the outer world. A given piece of
research, for example, may tell us something about slave life in
Virginia and attitudes toward illegitimacy; what we really know,
then, is something about slave life in Virginia and attitudes
toward illegitimacy; one must exercise the greatest care in
extending the geographical and time borders beyond the study,
whether from a laboratory or a piece of historical research.

In addition to the problems of external validity, however,

there are meaningful problems related to the internal validity of social science studies as well (Campbell, 1957, 1963). One of the factors which may interfere with obtaining satisfactory internal validity is a bias which is introduced by the researchers and their assistants, and which is inherently built into such studies (Rosenthal, 1963a, b, c, 1964). Researchers offer an hypothesis at the beginning of an experiment; the results of the experiment generally tend to confirm the hypothesis. An experimenter, because of his own biases, will tend to phrase questions or utilize inflections which convey a given intent to others participating in the experiment. Research assistants, even when not told the hypothesis in advance, usually figure out the experimenter's intent; they then collect data which tends to be supportive of the stated hypothesis. Even with researchers of marked sensitivity, this is a difficult problem to overcome.

A further source of difficulty is introduced by the subjects who participate in social science experiments. It has been shown quite convincingly that data collected from the reports of subjects tend to have built-in biases (Ore, 1962, 1964). Regardless of the subjects' motivations, most subjects will have some personal interpretation as to what the experiment is designed to prove. This interpretation may or may not be correct. Because of the interpretation, however, the subjects will make responses combining an interpretation of what the correct answer is, what the experiment is supposed to prove, and what the experimenter would like to hear, with the subjects' responses being further influenced by their like or dislike of the experimenter, and their view of what constitutes the goal of experiment (Seltiz, 1966).

Some studies have attempted to eliminate subject-introduced biases by utilizing unobtrusive measures (Webb, 1966). In this way, subjects are observed and studied without their awareness. Such studies raise questions concerning invasion of privacy, and are further not applicable for all types of data collection. Such measures may not be completely unobtrusive, so subject biases may still enter into the data collection. Researchers, however, should at least be cognizant of such techniques and should further be cognizant of subject biases (as well as researcher biases).

As would be expected, studies which have been reported in the literature concerning illegitimacy in general and teen-age pregnancies in specific have suffered from factors effecting both internal and external validity. Research has typically been carried out with a nonrandom sample of girls. Often it has been carried out by individuals who have special meaning in the girls' lives, meaning which could be expected to affect stated attitudes and aspirations. Conclusions have been drawn, and attempts have been made to generalize findings to all pregnant teen-agers.

Obviously, even if one ignores the serious questions relating to internal biases within the studies, the validity of widely generalizing from such data can be severely questioned. Individuals who are seen by a judge and court may be quite different from those who have no contact with the judicial system. Girls who receive no care may differ from those who are treated at public shelters, or who enter a maternity home. Girls who are referred to psychiatrists, especially when such referrals are made because of clinical indications, may be anticipated to have more emotional difficulties than those who neither receive such referrals nor are desirous of psychiatric help. Studies based upon lower socioeconomic, nonwhite pregnancies may deal with one set of issues. However, as has already been demonstrated in previous sections, the problems of the poor and of the nonwhite are not necessarily those of white middle-class society. Usually studies which generalize from observations made of the poor, the nonwhite, and the illegitimately pregnant girl, ignore the differences in backgrounds and needs between these girls and somewhat dissimilar individuals, and further ignore the whole population of predominantly white middle-class females who are similarly pregnant out of wedlock, but who get abortions, rather than carrying the pregnancies to term.

Another serious area of distortion may result from equating present day nonwhite attitudes with those of either a slave culture or a Caribbean society. One obviously does not equate the attitudes and temperaments of today's middle class housewives with those of women of fifty years ago. Nor does one equate today's women with southern belles of the 1800's, pioneer women of the early west, or inhabitants of primitive societies. Yet, with very little real evidence to support such claims, statements are made which closely link blacks today, at least attitudinally, with their ancestors who lived in very dissimilar societies. Such equations place too little emphasis upon the realities of the inner city: poverty, lack of opportunity, and relatively little mobility (Report of the National Advisory Commission on Civil Disorders, 1968).

At this time it is impossible to state that all pregnant teenagers are acting out for the same psychological reasons, although a psychological component may be an important factor in the pregnancies of a considerable number. Similarly, it is impossible to equate the etiology of all Negro and Puerto Rican unwed pregnancies with ancestral factors—although these factors may indeed have some limited significance. The more recent sociological orientation appears worthy of consideration. Where different meaning and values are emerging, where old traditions are shattering, and where sexual attitudes are markedly changing, premarital and extramarital intercourse, and, perhaps, out-of-wedlock pregnancies, may be more prevalent. Further, and of some importance, where there is physical overcrowding of families, where extreme poverty is present, where children have to demonstrate adult patterns of behavior in coping with the world from early ages, where anomie exists, and, where the meaning of adult success and opportunity has grossly different implications, the stage for early sexual activity and teen-age pregnancy may be set.

Again, as was true with medical problems, qualitatively and quantitatively the problems faced from a social service point of view may be related to age, socioeconomic background, race, illegitimacy, and other factors, such as psychological adjustment. It is important to recognize that differences, as well as similarities, may exist between individuals and between groups. Age alone is one factor. Age, compounded by the other parameters mentioned, may result in different problems for different girls. What, therefore, becomes increasingly important is that an awareness exists of the multiplicity of problems which pregnant teen-agers demonstrate from a social service point of view, and that sufficient, high quality services be available for these high-risk individuals.

THE SOCIAL SERVICES

As was true medically, once again one sees a high-risk group of individuals who, for a variety of reasons, have difficult problems which need to be solved. One may assume that those individuals of greatest risk will often have least mobility and least sophistication concerning the availability of services and opportunities to which they are entitled. One needs to identify the quality of services which are available to these teen-agers. One further needs to ask whether there is any differential of available services, and whether there is any differential of attitudes on the part of workers and agencies providing these services, which may be related to the background and problems presented by the pregnant girls.

Unfortunately, as has already been demonstrated medically, one quickly perceives that there is a differential of quality and quantity of services offered to those individuals who, at least within traditional sociological thinking, represent the highest risk. Services in general for pregnant teen-agers are inadequate. For the poor and for the nonwhite, they are particularly inadequate. In order to justify this claim, it seems appropriate to take a realistic and hard look at the types of services which various agencies and resources are providing.

A logical way to subdivide the existent social services is into three broad groups: those which occur in hospitals and clinics; those which are provided by voluntary agencies and homes for unwed mothers; and those which are provided by the community at large. An attempt will be made to review the extent, the availability, and the utilization of these services.

HOSPITALS AND CLINICS

Social service, as provided by hospitals, is considerably more limited than the general public would believe. In 1962, it was estimated that only fifteen percent of the hospitals in the United

States had social service departments (Herzog, 1964). Of these hospitals, many are staffed with extremely limited personnel, providing only superficial or screening services. Only a small proportion of hospitals offer even one social service contact for each unwed mother. And of these hospitals, the bulk are voluntary, rather than *clinic-oriented;* such voluntary hospitals serve a relatively small proportion of the unmarried mothers (Herzog, 1964). The rarity of adequate hospital social service for unmarried mothers becomes evident when one reviews the findings of the Community Council study involving New York City hospitals (Bernstein, 1963). In this study, 88 percent of the interviewed unmarried mothers had received their medical care through clinic types of facilities. Only 40 percent, however, had any contact with the clinic social worker. Of this minority which received any service, the bulk of the social service contacts appeared to be brief. Approximately one-third of all the contacts consisted of referrals to other agencies. Such referrals would usually be to community welfare departments for financial assistance, with little or no referral for counseling services. Only one-quarter of the women who received any hospital social service contact were given case work service. Thus, of the mothers interviewed in this large study, only 10 percent received what ordinarily would be defined as meaningful social service care.

VOLUNTARY AGENCIES AND HOMES FOR UNWED MOTHERS

Services provided by voluntary agencies, and especially homes for unwed mothers, are usually assumed by the public to be of major importance in answering the overall needs of the unwed mother. Many people are familiar with the meaningful effort made by Florence Crittendon and Booth Memorial Homes. What most do not realize is that such voluntary programs provide service for only a small minority of women pregnant out of wedlock. Further, the service tends to be limited by its nature to individuals of a markedly selected background. Maternity homes care for approximately 20,000 persons annually (Adams, 1963).

This is approximately 7 percent of the total population of unwed mothers. Patients who have insufficient mobility or knowledge of such services obviously would be unlikely to take advantage of them. Furthermore, the average fee for maternity home services is in excess of $750.00, and, as a result, individuals of low economic status are usually unable to apply. In addition, because of the orientation of homes and voluntary agencies, those individuals who are accepted for care usually have to meet the stipulation that they are planning to give the infants for adoption. As a result, most patients and certainly almost all nonwhite patients are excluded.

The financial requirements set by adoption agencies make it practically impossible for Negroes to qualify as adoptive parents. This means that a nonwhite girl who chooses to give her infant up for adoption could be fairly certain that no parents would be found. Further, interracial adoptions are not generally permitted through ordinary adoption channels, even if adoptive parents of a race other than that of the infant could be found. Therefore, in addition to other factors which make it difficult for a nonwhite or poor girl to enter a home for unwed mothers, there is the salient fact that she cannot give her child for adoption.

In spite of the figures which indicate that approximately 60 percent of the infants delivered out of wedlock are nonwhite, only 12 percent of the individuals cared for in maternity homes are nonwhite (Adams, 1963). As a result, not only must one regard studies from maternity homes as being applicable to only a small proportion of women pregnant out of wedlock, but one must realize that the services themselves benefit only a small segment of the population—usually white, middle class, mobile, and financially secure individuals who are planning on concealing their pregnancies.

THE COMMUNITY AT LARGE

Just as hospital and voluntary services tend to be inadequate and unavailable for the majority of those of highest medical risk, so, too, community sponsored programs are surprisingly inadequate. Rashbaum (1963) has reviewed the statistics for unmarried mothers receiving care at Mt. Sinai Hospital in New York City during 1956 and 1957. The results of this study are of significance as Mt. Sinai offers at least one social service contact to each unmarried mother in the clinic program. Of the 227 individuals participating in that study, the ethnic distribution was approximately 40 percent Negro, 30 percent white, and 30 percent Puerto Rican. Some biases were built into the study: the hospital is located in a predominantly Puerto Rican neighborhood; and the hospital tended to turn away women who had not registered for prenatal care by the seventh month of their pregnancy. Of the women studied, 27 percent were not known to any social agency other than the Mt. Sinai Hospital social service department. An additional 34 percent were known to only one other agency, that usually being the welfare department, where the individual was receiving financial assistance with little or no counseling. Only 39 percent of the women were receiving counseling.

When the figures were broken down by ethnic background, it was found that one white woman was not known to any social agency other than the hospital's social service department, and 13 percent were known to only one additional agency, usually the welfare department. The remaining 86 percent were known to two or more other social agencies. In addition, 85 percent of the white patients were known to a maternity home, and 38 percent were known also to a family service group. For other ethnic groups, marked differences were seen. Thirty-six percent of the Negro women were not known to any social agency other than that of the hospital, and 43 percent received service at only one other agency, usually the department of welfare. Only 21 percent were known to two or more outside social agencies. Of the Puerto Rican women, 44 percent were not known to any other agency, and an additional 44 percent were known to only one other agency, usually the department of welfare. Only 12 percent of Puerto Rican women received service from two or more agencies outside of the hospital.

A more recent study involving the greater Boston area in 1962 reports findings of a somewhat similar nature (Teele, 1967). Of the 1,335 women in the Boston study, 44.7 percent received

TABLE VIII

DISTRIBUTION OF SERVICES* RECEIVED BY UNMARRIED MOTHERS
WHO WERE PATIENTS AT MOUNT SINAI HOSPITAL, NEW YORK
DURING 1956–57—BY ETHNIC BACKGROUND OF MOTHERS

Number of Agencies Giving Service	Percent of Ethnic Group Receiving Services		
	Negro	White	Puerto Rican
No Agency	36	1	44
One Agency	43	13	44
Two Agencies	13	44	10
Three Agencies	5	34	2
Four or More Agencies	3	8	0

* In addition to the Mount Sinai Social Service Department
Abstracted from Rashbaum (1963)

no service from any social service agency during the period of study. Of those reported by agencies, one-third had no contacts other than those with hospital social service departments. Reported contacts with either family service agencies or the public welfare department were almost nonexistent.

Again, ethnic factors appeared to play a major role in determining the quantity and quality of social service care received. Forty-five percent of the white mothers had contact with maternity homes, child care agencies, or both; only 6 percent of black mothers had such contact. Eighty-one percent of the white mothers were known to some social agency within the community; only 11 percent of black mothers received such care. The relationships described appear to be independent of age. At every age level, substantially fewer black than white women had contact with child care agencies and/or maternity homes. For example, for those under twenty, over 50 percent of the white girls pregnant out of wedlock reported contacts with maternity homes, child care agencies, or both. Approximately 7 percent of Negroes reported similar care. One other factor which appeared to play a role in determining social service contact in the Boston study was parity of the mother. When the illegitimate pregnancy was a repeat, rather than a first experience, far fewer social service contacts existed. Once again, since repeat illegitimate pregnancies would tend to be more prevalent in the Negro

TABLE IX

PROPORTIONS OF UNWED MOTHERS IN BOSTON WHO HAD
REPORTED CONTACTS WITH MATERNITY HOMES, CHILD
CARE AGENCIES, OR BOTH DURING 1962 BY AGE
AND RACE OF MOTHERS

	Race				
	*White (N = 920)**			*Negro (N = 402)**	
Age	No.	%		No.	%
16 years and under	38	49.3	(77)	4	8.0	(50)
17—18 years	94	50.3	(187)	4	6.6	(61)
19 years	72	59.5	(121)	3	6.7	(45)
20—29 years	182	41.5	(439)	10	4.8	(208)
30 years and over	27	28.1	(96)	3	7.9	(38)

* Numbers on which proportions are based in parentheses
From Teele (1967)

and poor nonwhite population, such individuals would have even fewer social service contacts.

Since the majority of non-hospital contacts for clinic patients, especially for nonwhite clinic patients, are with social welfare departments, it seems worth looking at such contacts a little more closely. I have been unable to find the existence of significant counseling within welfare departments for these individuals. Where counseling exists, it is geared to mothers who are planning to surrender their infants; thus counseling is oriented to white females pregnant out of wedlock, and often it is further oriented towards middle-class white females who have contacted the welfare department in an attempt to make arrangements for future adoption. When any contact exists for nonwhite clients, it is almost always for the explicit purpose of determining and arranging financial assistance.

What one sees emerging, therefore, is a gross inequality of social service counseling for pregnant teen-agers, with the presence of adequate counseling being related to race, socioeconomic status, and decisions concerning possible surrender of the unborn infant. On a national basis, it has been estimated that only one out of six unwed mothers receives voluntary or public social service (Adams, 1963). This figure includes all women who are known to be pregnant out of wedlock. Obviously, for the more disadvantaged groups the figures would be markedly lower.

One may question the reasons for this lack of adequate counseling. Certainly an explanation may be related to societal attitudes which exist toward women who are pregnant out of wedlock. Although compassion and pity may be voiced, there are certainly smoldering feelings which condemn the involved individuals for their "immorality." It is this author's conviction that there further exists a relatively common desire on the part of "helping" officials to punish such individuals who are pregnant out of wedlock. Often, these feelings are thinly disguised. The persons who claim to be most involved with the welfare of girls pregnant out of wedlock may strongly oppose meaningful attempts to help the girls integrate themselves into the community at large rather than becoming traditional charity cases. More than occasionally one may hear the statement that things are being made too easy, or that the girl will not *learn* from her experience.

Perhaps it is possible to crystallize the notions of shame and disgrace as even existing in those areas where intensive service is offered, such as maternity homes. The girl leaves her community when the pregnancy becomes physically obvious. She is sheltered for the remainder of the pregnancy, often with little activity or education being available during this time. Following delivery, she surrenders the infant for adoption and, in many centers, has no contact with the infant during her stay in the hospital. She is told it is a mistake which has now been erased. One gets the feeling that she is sent home, supposedly having purified herself and having become absolved of her "sins." Many maternity homes advise the girls not to communicate with them in the future. Further, an explicit statement may be made that if another pregnancy occurs out of wedlock, it will not be viewed as an accident, and the girl will not be welcome to return for care. As one thinks through these concepts, it certainly becomes difficult to divorce the attitudes of the personnel from those of a group of judges sentencing, condemning, and finally absolving a hardened criminal. A moral judgment is inherently conveyed.

Although the girls may be told that they are bringing a new life into the world, that this life is itself good, and that the girls themselves are not necessarily bad individuals, it would be indeed surprising if the very actions, behaviors, and orientation of the personnel did not send out strong messages to the contrary. The girl who is confined to such an institution, separated from family and friends, excluded from school, employment, and meaningful activities, and forbidden to communicate with the institution if she again becomes pregnant, would certainly understand the attitude of those helping her, and the expectation for her to repent and emerge cleansed.

With lower socioeconomic girls, and especially nonwhite girls, still different conditions and attitudes prevail. These girls, on the whole, do not conceal their pregnancies. They do not leave their homes. The community in which they live knows of their pregnancy. The girls even keep and raise the future child.

Such behavior tends to provoke a variety of reactions in the white middle-class population. Not uncommonly one may hear a type of praise for the permissive, non-condemning, black community. A general attitude prevails which states that the Negro community does not condemn illegitimacy. Pregnancy out of wedlock is allegedly no cause for shame. Such an attitude can find historical comfort from the previously-mentioned studies which point to the descent from slavery of Negro culture. It is pointed out that the Negro family is matriarchal, often with no significant or even present male in the household. Sexual freedom occurs from an earlier age, and pregnancy is the inevitable, and not unexpected, result.

One does not have to be extremely astute to perceive condescension and bigotry in such attitudes. Perhaps there indeed is some degree of carry-over from the mores of slave culture. However, the continuous emphasis upon such historical and anthropological data undoubtedly reflects deeper feelings which may not be as easily spoken. Just as the social distance between medical personnel and patient caused alienation and created medical care problems, similarities can be found in the social service situation. Along with any anthropological and cultural claims obviously go further interpretations. One such interpretation concerns Negro morality and the commonly held notion that the Negro is more sexually promiscuous, more sexually potent, and more socially amoral. Whenever differences are stressed, one may further wonder if there is also implicit judgment concerning the ability of the Negro to assume meaningful roles in a white middle-class society. Although it does not necessarily follow, the question may even be asked as to whether the emphasis upon anthropological and cultural data may be a technique of alluding to the notion of Negro cultural inferiority, and even to the equating of the American Negro with a savage who must be protected by the more capable and learned members of society.

A COMMENT ON ATTITUDES

In carefully reviewing the literature, the author has been unable to find any proof of widespread differences in the black population in the United States today which would condone or encourage out-of-wedlock pregnancy in teen-agers, or in any other members of the group. There have been no studies which demonstrate pride in the out-of-wedlock condition in a significant number of individuals, or lack of concern for the educational consequences to the mother, or for the responsibility which the pregnancy will bring to the family. Where data is available, which deals with the meaning of out-of-wedlock pregnancy to families with social mobility and with desires for educational and job improvement (or even when data is available for less mobile families), the inferences are quite to the contrary (Bernard, 1966; Hertz, 1944; Himes, 1964; Osili, 1957).

Some obvious problems have been ignored in the literature. The most striking of these problems concerns the area of adoption. As has been mentioned, it has been commonly assumed that nonwhite mothers do not place infants for adoption because of family acceptance of illegitimacy, and even pride and love for the unborn child. Perhaps such acceptance and ability to display love and pride are more common with the Negro population. It is possible that the traditions of the white middle-class population tend to discourage such feelings.

However, another important explanation exists for the paucity of nonwhite adoptions; this by necessity must account for a considerable number of nonwhite mothers who decide to keep their offspring. The explanation rests upon one of the facts of present day life: there are almost no adoptive homes for nonwhite children. This situation is true throughout the country. Few nonwhite families can qualify as prospective parents under the present traditional state requirements. Their incomes may not be sufficiently high by middle-class standards. The size and layout of the living facilities are often inadequate by middle-class standards. Parental education may be lacking; the mother may work part or full time, a situation disapproved of by welfare departments. These factors tend to disqualify prospective parents. One-parent homes are not even considered in many states at this time (although an increasing number of cases of one-parent adoptions are occurring, with children given to both single men and single women). The same difficulties are present, although to a different degree, when foster home placement is considered. Parents who might be adequate can often not meet the qualifications of the welfare departments. Further, in the case of foster home placement, remuneration is often grossly inadequate and few attempts are made to recruit, or to assist those who might be excellent and warm prospective parents to obtain the necessary requirements.

One additional problem should not be overlooked. For the average nonwhite family in this country, welfare workers have a distinctly negative connotation. They have traditionally been thought of as serving not in the client's interest, but rather in the interest of the welfare department. Poor people often worry about the meaning of the visit of a welfare worker. What will the worker discover? Will a violation be uncovered which will lead to the discontinuation of welfare checks? Even when violations are not discovered, workers have attempted to interfere with the family functioning and have insisted upon changes in purchasing or in utilizing materials. This is understandably resented by the recipients. With adoptions and adoption evaluations being frequently linked to welfare departments, and with the possibility of intensive investigation by workers, it is not surprising that few nonwhite individuals offer themselves as prospective adoptive parents.

Just as the issue of adoption becomes almost nonexistent for the nonwhite pregnant teen-ager, so, too, other traditional social services areas become more difficult. Without the alternative of possible adoption, maternity homes demonstrate relatively little concern for the problems of the nonwhite teen-ager. Further, the nonwhite individual tends to be excluded from such maternity home service because of relative inability to pay. With the average nonwhite family income in this country being far below that of the average white family, relatively few nonwhite individuals can afford the costs of maternity home care. There would, in addition, be some individuals in the nonwhite community who, because of lack of knowledge of available facilities and care, would have insufficient background to allow them to take advantage of even those minimal facilities which would be readily available to them.

Because of the unavailability of adoptive homes for nonwhite children, counseling, even when present, has been very different for the nonwhite mother than it is for the white mother. Although claims may be made that all girls, regardless of race or background, can receive equal counseling and are free to make independent decisions, one may question whether this is true. When workers know that no adoptive homes are available, they are unlikely to allow girls to give vent to any positive feelings about adoption. As a result, welfare workers have traditionally encouraged nonwhite clients to keep their babies, and, because of financial reasons, have often encouraged teen-age girls to remain at home after the birth of the infant to care for it, rather than returning to school. Obviously, this type of advice is different from what would be given to a white, pregnant teen-ager. Perhaps related to the combination of biases which exist within the traditional middle-class agencies, and socioeconomic and adoptive problems which uniquely exist for the nonwhite population, the traditional counseling for such clients, when existent, has consisted of helping the individual to meet financial and living facility problems. It is no wonder that the figures reported from studies, such as those from Boston (Teele, 1967), and New York

(Rashbaum, 1963), demonstrate a relative paucity of social service counseling for nonwhite, pregnant individuals.

Thus, one can easily see that a paradox exists. The white, middle-class girl who is concealing her infant and planning for future adoption receives the most intensive social service care. In addition, this girl tends to have more financial and community support. Her medical care is often better and the medical prognosis both for her and for her unborn child is better than that which exists for other groups. This girl, who starts off with the most favored prognosis, receives the highest quality of care.

On the other hand, poor and especially nonwhite individuals who, from a social service point of view are at highest risk, receive the least adequate counseling and assistance. These are the girls whose living conditions are most crowded, whose diets are least adequate, whose medical prognosis is most guarded, and, who, in addition, either by choice or necessity are going to be left with the responsibility at a young age of caring for a future offspring. It would seem that social service counseling would have much to offer this population. Attempts could be made to help the girls seek out more adequate medical care to prevent complications for themselves and their babies. Efforts could be made to provide adoptive homes in order that these girls at least be given the options which are at present available to their white middle-class peers. Even if this option is absent, however, other areas of counseling are obviously necessary: techniques of infant care, adjustment to society, and possible future education are all of major significance.

The pregnant teen-ager must definitely be considered at high risk from a social service point of view. More adequate counseling must be made available for all pregnant teen-agers; they must also be made aware of the existence of counseling. For white, middle-class pregnant teen-agers there are areas of gross deficiency and inadequacy. These certainly need to be remedied. However, even a more acute paucity of services is available for the poor, and especially the nonwhite. Attempts must be made to offer meaningful services to these individuals if a realistic integration into society is to be expected either from them or their offspring.

IV

THE EDUCATIONAL PROBLEM

We have read that the pregnant teen-ager does indeed represent a medical and social service high risk individual. From an educational point of view, therefore, a similar question must be asked. Is the pregnant teen-ager at high risk educationally? The answer is obvious and definite: Yes.

It is easy to hypothesize the extent of the educational problem. Motherhood, in marriage or without it, is bound to interrupt education, unless adequate child care facilities are provided by the society. In this country, only recently has the need for child care centers been getting the attention it has deserved for years. At the federally-sponsored level, some child care facilities are being set up for the poor. Hopefully, these will be professionally and adequately staffed; hopefully also, such facilities will go beyond the poverty communities.

Although these child care centers may change the situation, today welfare workers are urging their recipients to stay home with their children. This means that a fifteen-year-old girl who conceives an illegitimate infant is *counseled* to discontinue her education. Needless to say, a meaningful future for her is severely hampered by such counseling.

The problem of defining the degree of educational risk facing the pregnant teen-ager is not an easy one, however. Not only have relatively few studies been done, but those which have been reported have faced serious obstacles. It has not been an easy task to isolate or define the number of pregnant teen-agers who exist at any one time in any given community. The reasons for the difficulty must be obvious to the reader. Discrepancies exist in reports concerning teen-agers from the middle class, as opposed to those from the low socioeconomic class. In order to

60

avoid community knowledge of an existing pregnancy, a middle-class girl's parents may obtain a physician's certificate claiming that the girl must leave school for a variety of medical reasons, such as exhaustion, debilitation, or mononucleosis. School authorities, while often cognizant of false excuses, tend to support the girl's desire for secrecy, and, as a result, do not question such excuses. Therefore, any data gathering which utilizes school records as source material has a built-in bias which excludes middle-class teen-age pregnancies. As a result, the proportion of lower socioeconomic, and, especially, nonwhite pregnancies, is overemphasized.

The problems which arise when one attempts to make this data-collecting more accurate are numerous. Not only are school records inaccurate, with biases concerning middle-class girls, but other sources of information often do not correct for this inaccuracy. Medical ethics and standards of confidentiality tend to assist a number of girls in keeping their pregnancies from becoming known. Family pressures and influence may similarly contribute to an individual's successfully concealing her pregnancy. As has previously been mentioned, even when one utilizes birth certificate information, these difficulties cannot be fully overcome. Birth certificates cannot, of course, give meaningful statistics about illegal abortion. Nor can such information account for individuals who use pseudonyms or claim marriage to avoid the stigma of an out-of-wedlock pregnancy. It would seem, therefore, that, although one can gain considerable information concerning the relationship of the pregnant teen-ager to education, one must realize from the onset that there are certain inherent difficulties which limit available data.

In spite of the inaccuracies in reporting school exclusion due to pregnancy, some meaningful and important information has become available. The data reported from Maryland (Stine, 1964), demonstrates that pregnancy is the most frequent physical condition causing an adolescent to leave school prior to graduation. More than twice as many adolescent females leave school because of the diagnosis of pregnancy than for all other medical and physical conditions put together. The experience in Maryland can probably be generalized to the remainder of the country. As has already been reported, the absolute number of teen-age pregnancies has been rising throughout the country. In addition, however, there has been an increasing awareness of the prevalence and importance of this problem. As a result, school health officials during the past several years have noted a marked increase in the number of girls leaving school due to pregnancy. Part of this increase can be accounted for by the rising number of school-age girls who become pregnant each year. The remainder of the rise can probably be related to the belated interest shown this problem by school officials. Whatever the reasons, there is no question but that almost every school system in the country has noted the magnitude of the problem and its relationship to school dropout.

PREGNANCY AND THE SCHOOL SYSTEM

One must raise serious questions concerning school policy throughout the country in reference to pregnant teen-agers. With relatively few exceptions, the policy of school boards has been to *exempt* from attendance girls who are pregnant when their condition becomes obvious or, in the judgment of the school principal, is detrimental to the individual or to the morale of the school. Not only has this been the policy of individual school boards, but often this thinking has become generalized as state-wide policy (Burchind, 1960; Derthick, 1960; Kelley, 1963; Murdock, 1967). Most school boards have then had the policy of continuing the exclusion until after adoption of the newborn infant or until after adequate plans are made for infant care, if the mother plans to keep her infant; and going a step further, some boards have mandated permanent school exclusion, regardless of plans for the infant.

In general, judicial decisions have upheld the validity of such school board interpretations. The reasons cited include the supposed influence of a girl's pregnancy upon her own performance and the morale of other students; the physical well-being of the expectant mother is also given as a justification (Welfare Law Bulletin, 1968). One may ask, what is the implication of such policy? Most educators have used such policy and court decision to exclude girls from school as soon as the pregnancy is known. There are exceptions where girls are allowed to remain in school for longer periods of time, but these exceptions are in the distinct minority.

For the middle-class girl, who is planning to conceal the pregnancy and place her infant for adoption, this approach may result in six-to-nine month exclusion from school. For the lower socioeconomic girl, and especially the nonwhite girl, who is neither concealing the pregnancy nor placing her infant for adoption, the exclusion from school may be for a period of up to eighteen months. The reason for this high figure is that often nine months postpartal go by before the girl is adjudged to have made adequate plans for care of her infant.

The impression has definitely been gathered that middle-class girls, on the whole, remain in school for a longer period of time prior to exclusion. It at least seems that middle-class girls are kept in school for several months when the pregnancy is not grossly obvious, and until the girl is ready to leave for a maternity home. The lower socioeconomic girl, especially if nonwhite, seems to be excluded from school at an earlier date.

Just as previous sections have demonstrated the biases of medical and social service personnel towards lower socioeconomic individuals, similar biases undoubtedly exist within school systems. In the inner-city schools, where students have not consistently demonstrated middle-class motivation as desired by school personnel, and where parents have neither the status nor the relationships with teachers which are enjoyed by middle-class parents, the teachers and principal may have little desire to keep a girl in school as long as possible. Just as physicians offer less adequate care to such individuals, and just as welfare workers encourage pregnant teen-agers of lower socioeconomic status to remain at home after the birth of their infants, showing little regard for the future mother's needs and potentialities, so, too, school officials may often not be totally displeased with the girl's dropout from school. This is especially true if the girl has been "an under-achiever." School officials know that if a girl is out of school for eighteen months, it is unlikely that she will return, because of both the long interruption and her past history. Even if she does return, her chances for success are extremely remote. An Illinois study (Hoeft, 1968) has demonstrated that over half of such girls drop out of school again within one year with poor records of attendance and a relatively high percentage of delinquency. Therefore, it would not be surprising to see school officials actually encouraging earlier departure from school.

The author has gained the impression that the girls who need education most—those who have had the most difficulty obtaining a satisfactory educational relationship in the past, and who have the least opportunity for meaningful employment or role in the community in the future without further education—are the girls who are most likely to be excluded from school early in the pregnancy. They are further most likely to be excluded from school for longer periods of time following the delivery of their infants.

THE REASONS FOR SCHOOL EXCLUSION

One, of course, must logically question the rationale of excluding girls from school at all because of pregnancy. The stated reasons include the impact of the pregnancy upon the girl and her ability to function in a school situation, and the impact of the obvious pregnancy at a later point upon her fellow students. One must question the wisdom of this reasoning: are these rational interpretations meaningful in themselves, or are they cover-ups for individual biases, and for puritanical moral judgments?

First of all, one may medically ask what there is about a pregnancy which would interfere with normal carrying out of school function. Most physicians allow patients full activity and employment opportunity throughout a pregnancy, unless complications supervene. One could certainly wonder why these same judgments could not be made for the pregnant teen-ager. If medical complications occurred, certainly the individual would require treatment. She could then be excused from school medically as would any other individual with a medical problem. If no complications arose, there would be no medical reason to exclude the girl from school. It is difficult to understand why any pregnant girl without medical problems could not remain, if she so desired, within her school until the onset of labor, and why she further could not return to school within a couple weeks following the delivery of her infant. There are many illnesses which result in student's leaving school for longer periods of time without penalty. There are certainly other medical conditions which can result in more medical jeopardy while attending school than pregnancy. At the present time, such illnesses do not appear to interfere with regular school attendance.

If the girl is not being excluded from school because of detriment to herself as an individual, one may then wonder why the pregnant teen-ager is excluded from school at all. The second part of the reason is usually that the girl should be excluded from school because her pregnancy is detrimental to the morale of the school. One may ask how one girl's pregnancy can be detrimental to the morale of the school. To assume that the pregnancy is detrimental to the morale of other teen-agers requires a certain line of thinking. It is the thinking that "one bad apple spoils the bushel of apples."

It must be assumed that other girls in the classroom, seeing the example of the one or two pregnant teen-agers, would themselves decide to become pregnant. Pregnancy would soon become so rampant that all classrooms would be full of pregnant teenagers. Obviously such thinking is fallacious. If anything, since most teen-agers are more altruistic than their parents or other adults, one might well wonder if the existence of pregnant teenagers in classrooms would have just the opposite effect. Sensitive teen-agers, exposed to the reality of the problems facing the peer who had become pregnant at an early age, at a time when she was not ready for the responsibilities of motherhood, might in fact be deterred from early pregnancy and early marriage. It is not considered inappropriate for teen-agers to learn about problems in the political arena; they also study about health problems and other problems related to adult life. Parents and school officials might even feel that students would benefit from being exposed to individuals with difficulty; the compassion and understanding which would develop would be of help to them throughout their lives.

Part of the reason for hiding pregnancy must lie in a conscious or unconscious puritanism in our country. Pregnant teachers are excluded early in their pregnancies from the schools, on ostensible grounds that it is for their own health. A quick second reason is that the children would ask questions about the condition, and thus, sex education might have to begin. Since most children see their mothers pregnant, or at least see the neighbors pregnant, this reason is a mockery. To many teachers, such exclusion presents an economic hardship, since maternity leaves are without pay.

It sounds illogical indeed to suggest that pregnant teachers and students are excluded from school because we are trying to forget the sexual facts of life—particularly since these facts are made so graphic by the mass media—but such may be the case.

Another reason for excluding the pregnant adolescent from school is our general confusion over teen-age drives and responsibilities. There exists some myth that, if left to his own devices, every teen-age boy would be madly seducing every teen-age girl. This state of affairs would be further compounded by the teenage girl, who, in accordance with the myth of woman as witchlike seductress of men, would lead all the boys to their destruction. One must wonder about the unrealistic and unsatisfactory state of adult sexuality, that would permit such ideas to flourish.

These ideas would suggest that years of parental and community efforts directed towards making children responsible citizens have no effect. They further would suggest that human beings, and especially females, have no motivations, desires, and feelings of a nonsexual nature. To think thus would certainly be a very superficial dismissal of humanity.

Another, and perhaps even more distressing, aspect of society's exclusion of pregnant teen-agers from school is one which is even less explicitly stated. Since there can be no philosophical or intellectual justification for the excuse of protecting the girls and of further protecting the sensitivities of their classmates, one is compelled to ask whether the adults who enforce such decisions are indeed trying to hurt and punish the pregnant girl. This certainly would not be the first episode in the history of mankind in which groups of people, claiming that their actions were based upon moral and righteous fervor, have discriminated against, and even persecuted, others. Certainly, if one traces the history of womanhood, it is not difficult to find many examples where women have been held in a grossly subservient and difficult role by the remainder of society. When women have deviated at all from the roles prescribed for them, punishment has followed. Even when women have not deviated from anticipated roles, they still have at times been subject to unrealistic punishment, such as existed during the time when women were sentenced as, and even executed for, being witches.

The educational, judicial, and social decisions which exclude pregnant teen-agers from school are nothing more than harshly punitive and unjust. There is a thinly disguised set of punitive feelings which desire to shame, disgrace, and hurt the adolescent for her misbehavior. She is to be burned at the stake like the witches of old in order that others may benefit from her punishment. It is hoped that other teen-agers will refrain from sexual activity after seeing what society's punishment is for a pregnant girl. In the name of protection the girl is excluded from school. Society criticizes her for living on welfare roles, and yet she is excluded from possible education which would allow her to have a meaningful role as an adult, and, perhaps, as a result, to keep off the welfare roles.

Instead of regarding teen-age pregnancy as a situation for which the individual is perhaps unready, the pregnancy is regarded as a crime. Instead of seeing the pregnant teen-ager as being an individual who, if anything, is in need of more help and understanding by society at a time of crisis in her life, the girl is treated as a criminal to be shunned, one who may return to society only if she purges herself of her guilt and is fully remorseful.

THE EDUCATIONAL BACKGROUNDS OF
PREGNANT STUDENTS

It seems appropriate to briefly look at the information which is available concerning the educational background of students who become pregnant during adolescence. The data is distinctly limited and biased. The more favored middle- and upper-class girls, who are able to conceal their pregnancies from school authorities, or whose favored position within the community results in the authorities' not questioning the reason for their prolonged absences from school, do not usually get into the data. Since they "are not pregnant," and since their names cannot be listed in the school registers concerning out-of-wedlock mothers, information concerning them is sparse. Further, those girls who enter maternity homes or other types of shelters, at least are offered some type of education.

It is the poor, and especially the nonwhite, pregnant teen-ager who not only is available for most complete study but who is the individual most excluded from any educational, social, and medical advantages which society has to offer. Among those groups who are unprotected from prying investigations, and who are thus unable to retain anonymity—the poor, and especially the nonwhite—the available figures indicate a high incidence of teen-age pregnancy, and, therefore, a high incidence of school and future educational exclusion. The previously mentioned Maryland figures indicate that 2.6 percent of fourteen-year-old, 7.5 percent of fifteen-year-old, and 13.6 percent of sixteen-year-old Negro girls are pregnant (Stine, 1964). These may sound like astoundingly high figures. If one could include abortions and hidden pregnancies in middle- and upper-class families, the figures, while being somewhat different, would not be markedly dissimiliar. This information, combined with the further information which adds that 20 percent of the sixteen-year-old pregnancies are not first pregnancies, shows the overwhelming magnitude of the problem.

Pakter's (1961a) study of New York City births during 1955-59 included data from the Bureau of Attendance of the New York City Board of Education concerning 259 cases of pregnancy among girls who were, at the time of pregnancy, attending school. Confirming previous statements which have claimed that the girls who most frequently are included in large community studies are those from lower socioeconomic and nonwhite groups, because of absence of mobility and the type of power which insures anonymity, the ethnic distribution was 69.5 percent Negro,

17 percent Puerto Rican, and 11.2 percent white. Only 4 percent of the girls were stated to have poor relationships with their peers or siblings, and a relatively small number, 13 percent, were reported as having poor relationships with their parents. As might be expected from any study, and especially an inner-city type of study, 9 percent of the girls were reported as being in poor health; 12 percent were reported as being behavior problems; two-thirds of the girls came from broken homes.

One of the more striking and easily misused statistics in the study related to the I.Q. test scores of this group. The scores revealed that about one-third had an I.Q. of less than 75. Another one-third tested with an I.Q. of 75-90. Only one-third were classified within the traditionally normal limits, with an I.Q. of 90 or over. Only two girls in the entire group had an I.Q. of 125 or higher. About 50 percent of the girls had a prior history of truancy and had been reported as having an unfavorable attitude toward education.

As has been stated, this data may be of considerable importance to the serious investigator. The danger, however, is that this type of information tends to be easily misconstrued and utilized to the detriment of the individuals who are represented in this study. The scores and background information certainly indicate educational difficulty from the traditional point of view. The girls for the most part would be nonachievers within the classroom framework. There is an appropriate implication that such students would not thrive or significantly contribute to the progress of a traditional, and especially suburban, white middle-class classroom. This would be especially true at the time when the measurements and evaluations were taken. Such information, if improperly utilized, could be further ammunition for those who wish to punish and exclude pregnant girls from classrooms. Factors such as *lack of motivation, truancy,* and *low I.Q.* can be used to aid those who wish to formulate a morally justifiable policy of exclusion.

Such thinking unfortunately fails to take into account the real issues which the above data should illustrate. The girls, who would be available for such research efforts, are from the inner-city. On the whole, they are Negro and Puerto Rican. Poor health would certainly be expected within this population. Broken homes would also be predicted in a population riddled by poverty and anomie (Glick, 1963). Truancy and behavior disorders in school again are anticipated in areas where the population is extremely poor and nonwhite (Chilman, 1965).

Further, available knowledge has strongly demonstrated that I.Q. scores, school achievement, and school dropout can be directly correlated with such background dimensions (Burkhead, 1967; Coleman, 1966; *Daedalus*, 1965; Fine, 1967; Frost, 1966; Hughson, 1964; Pettigrew, 1964; Yourman, 1964).

Nationally, it has been well demonstrated that Negro children fare less well in school systems. They score lower in all standard tests of achievement; as they progress in school they fall farther behind the norms for their grade levels; here the effects of differential education are all too apparent (Coleman, 1966).

Familial background, parental support, parental education and occupation, exposure to similar items, language difficulties, and other factors too numerous to mention, all critically affect I.Q. scores and achievement (Deutsch, 1967). In New York City, intelligence scores have been found to be significantly lower among nonwhite and low socioeconomic grade school students than for white and more affluent students (Whiteman, 1967). Studies reported from Atlanta and Chicago, by Burkhead (1967), have shown strongly negative correlations between I.Q. in the ninth and eleventh grades and both nonwhite and low socioeconomic backgrounds. Low family income, especially, has strongly correlated with persistent low I.Q. scores and school dropout. In Syracuse, the results have been similar (Personal Communication, 1968). Children in inner-city schools have I.Q. and achievement measures which are considerably lower than those of children in middle-class neighborhoods. By grade 3, the average students in the inner-city school is already one year below grade level. This differential is not made up as the years go on. Perhaps, in less than a facetious manner, it has been suggested that I.Q. tests be utilized as a measure of socioeconomic background, rather than of intelligence.

Utilizing socioeconomic, ethnic, and cultural data to better understand the meaning of low I.Q. test results is not meant to

TABLE X

VERBAL ABILITY: NUMBER OF STANDARD DEVIATIONS BELOW
AND NUMBER OF GRADE LEVELS BEHIND THE AVERAGE
WHITE IN METROPOLITAN NORTHEAST, FOR ALL
GROUPS IN THE UNITED STATES

	Standard Deviation Below			*Grade Levels Behind*		
Grade of Student	6	9	12	6	9	12
White, nonmetropolitan:						
South	0.4	0.5	0.5	0.7	1.0	1.5
Southwest	.2	.2	.2	.3	.4	.8
North	.1	.2	.3	.2	.4	.9
White, metropolitan:						
Northeast	—	—	—	—	—	—
Midwest	.1	.0	.1	.1	.0	.4
South	.3	.2	.3	.5	.5	.9
Southwest	.3	.3	.2	.5	.6	.7
West	.2	.1	.1	.3	.3	.5
Negro, nonmetropolitan:						
South	1.5	1.7	1.9	2.5	3.9	5.2
Southwest	1.3	1.5	1.7	2.0	3.3	4.7
North	1.2	1.2	1.4	1.9	2.7	4.2
Negro, metropolitan:						
Northeast	1.0	1.1	1.1	1.6	2.4	3.3
Midwest	1.0	1.0	1.1	1.7	2.2	3.3
South	1.3	1.4	1.5	2.0	3.0	4.2
Southwest	1.2	1.4	1.5	1.9	2.9	4.3
West	1.2	1.2	1.3	1.9	2.6	3.9
Mexican American	1.3	1.1	1.1	2.0	2.3	3.5
Puerto Rican	1.7	1.3	1.2	2.7	2.9	3.6
Indian American	1.1	1.0	1.1	1.7	2.1	3.5
Oriental American	.6	.4	.5	.9	1.0	1.6

From Coleman (1966)

TABLE XI

IQ SCORES BY RACE AND SOCIOECONOMIC BACKGROUND
IN NEW YORK STUDY

Group	*Mean IQ Scores*
Socioeconomic Group I (Lowest)	94.31
Socioeconomic Group II (Middle)	102.67
Socioeconomic Group III (Highest)	109.16
Negro	97.01
White	106.08

Abstracted from Whiteman (1967)

TABLE XII

CORRELATIONS OF SOCIOECONOMIC VARIABLES AND SELECTED
TEST SCORES—22 ATLANTA PUBLIC HIGH SCHOOLS*

	Scores	
	8th Grade IQ	*10th Grade Verbal*
Median Family Income	.81	.79
Education of Adults	.90	.85
Percentage Nonwhite	—.90	—.89
Percentage White Collar	.90	.89
Percentage Deteriorated and Dilapidated Housing	—.87	—.85

* Correlation values that exceed .49 are significant at the .01 level.
Abstracted from Burkhead (1967)

imply that inner-city students do not present significant difficulties from the educator's point of view. Such an attitude would obviously be naive. Poverty, broken homes, and anomie do not lead to scholarly excellence. Children who have had to cope with serious and adult problems of survival rather than with intellectual endeavors, from an early age often have less interest in school activities. Truancy and behavior disorders are not problems which can be treated easily by school systems. The low I.Q. scores, while not necessarily reflecting inferior intelligence, reflect real problems in student educability, given the

TABLE XIII

CORRELATIONS OF SOCIOECONOMIC VARIABLES AND SELECTED
TEST SCORES—39 CHICAGO PUBLIC HIGH SCHOOLS*

	IQ Scores	
	9th Grade	*11th Grade*
Median Family Income	.92	.90
Education of Adults	.57	.59
Percentage Nonwhite	—.86	—.84
Percentage White Collar	.70	.75
Percentage Substandard Housing	—.79	—.74

* Correlation values that exceed .40 are significant at the .01 level.
Abstracted from Burkhead (1967)

present limits in education. For whatever reason the scores may be low, they indicate that these students are not thriving within the traditional classrooms. They are not achieving at the rates prescribed for middle-class students. They are falling behind in school work, and have either failed many semesters, or have been advanced merely because the system does not know how else to respond to such students. The educational difficulties are staggering and, at times, even overwhelming.

SOME EDUCATIONAL QUESTIONS

However, the author asserts that pregnant teen-agers should not be excluded from school. Their prior failure to thrive within the traditional school system has a variety of etiologic explanations (Bernard, 1942, 1966; Chilman, 1965; Glick, 1963; Putnam, 1963; Tamber, 1964). Family structure, parental attitudes, and individual motivation all play a role. Society, however, also plays a significant role. Society contributes to student failure because of long-standing persecution and discrimination which have influenced both parental and student aspiration and ability to achieve. Society also contributes to inner-city failure through its treatment of such children prior to any delinquency, and certainly prior to any pregnancy. Inner-city children are high-risk students. Yet, just as the poor, high-risk medical patients are treated less as patients and more as undesirable, lower-class human beings, and just as such clients are treated as stereotypes and caricatures of a formerly existent southern slave culture by social agencies, educationally one sees a similarly deplorable situation.

Inner-city students with language, familial, assimilation, and economic difficulties are at highest risk educationally. Not only to stimulate these children but to assist them in a struggle to achieve within an alien society necessitates a meaningful and extensive effort by the school systems. When children begin with distrust of their teachers, who to them represent the middle-class hostile world, when children have difficulty communicating with a white, middle-class dialect, when children's orientation is that regardless of education, jobs will not be available, when children's families have not set standards of educational excellence, when overcrowding, lack of food and real difficulty in survival all exist—the conditions for school failure, delinquency, and low achievement all exist.

To assist such individuals in aiding themselves requires a major effort. From the very beginning, educational tools must be exciting and meaningful. Teachers must be sensitive and abundant. Conditions must be optimal.

These have not been the answers provided by the school system and by society at large. White, middle-class, suburban children of motivated, achievement-oriented parents can succeed in almost any school system. Inner-city children need, if anything, much more attention and effort if progress is to be made. Yet, the offered answers have not taken these facts into consideration. The worst schools are the inner-city schools. The pupil-teacher ratios are highest. Physcial facilities, atheletic facilities, books and learning aids are worst. The students who need least get the most from the school systems, and the students who need most are given least. It is the pattern which is seen over and over again.

Simple answers to this problem are difficult to find. Education is financed from public funds. The middle and upper classes, therefore, contribute the bulk of the money for public education (it should be noted, however, that the poor contribute proportionately more of their income), although they frequently do not avail themselves of this education in inner-city areas. The more affluent persons in society have fewer children. If they dwell in the inner city area of urban centers, they often send their children to private schools. Because of the costs, the more affluent city dwellers typically want as little spent on public education as possible until riot and upheaval are at the back door—at which time they cry out for school reform, individualized instruction, and the upgrading of the inner-city school.

The point which seems to be overlooked is that the expenditure of more funds upon the education of the poor need not interfere with middle- and upper-class achievement. Giving assistance to one group in order that its members may lead more meaningful and productive lives does not by necessity result in less meaningful and productive lives for the remainder of the population. Equality of opportunity does not negate individual achievement or success. If anything, a society in which all members have greater opportunity would be likely to result in still further success and achievement for its members. There is room at the top for many.

With this in mind, implications of present-day policy toward pregnant teen-agers becomes unfortunately all too clear. A group of individuals with a past history of under-achievement, difficulty in adjustment, and even truancy, who are often performing considerably below stated grade level, are excluded from school. This exclusion, which is couched in humane terms, may be for a period of one and one-half years. If one takes a group of individuals who are already demonstrating little motivation, lack of achievement, and even delinquency, and excludes them from school for one and one-half years so that their level of performance is still farther behind that expected for individuals of their age, it is unrealistic to expect these individuals to return to school. It is even more unrealistic to expect them to return to school with greater motivation than before. When one compounds this difficulty with the encouragement by welfare workers for the girls to leave school and stay home in order to provide infant care, one has set the stage for large numbers of teen-age girls never returning to school.

Pregnant teen-agers should not be excluded from school. Especially in lower socioeconomic areas they are, if anything, already behind the expected grade level for their age group. Rather than exclusion, more help is needed. Schooling, counseling, and guidance should be intensified. Optional day care centers should be provided to make the attainment of education easier. Society, as well as the girls, can only benefit from keeping pregnant teen-agers in school. By having more education, by having a more realistic appraisal of meaningful values, and by further learning individual responsibility, pregnant teen-agers can become more fulfilled adults, better mothers, and better citizens.

The present educational ground rules for pregnant teen-agers are detrimental not only to lower socioeconomic girls, but to middle- and upper-class girls as well. The opportunities for wealthier girls are obviously not as restrictive. Maternity homes and other facilities often give some education. Further, since the pregnancy is hidden, it does not jeopardize the girl upon her return to school. She can return at an earlier date, because of placing the infant for adoption, and does not fall as far behind in her school work. If the pregnancy has been well hidden, she may not even have to suffer the social stigma of having been pregnant out of wedlock and of having to publicly acknowledge the pregnancy. But for these girls, too, the educational milieu is made difficult.

Most maternity homes provide less education than is imagined by the general public. A New York State survey revealed that the maximal education provided by maternity homes within that state consists of the availability of a teacher for one to two half-days per week (Lawrence, 1965). Even this limited educational program is the exception rather than the rule. The majority of homes provide no education whatsoever for the girls in attendance. There is no evidence to suggest that the situation is different in other states throughout the country. Thus, unless a girl is unusually motivated, education comes to a virtual standstill during this long period of time.

The effects of this educational compromise are added to the guilt and fear which already exist within the girl. If she is to return to school, she faces the prospect of being four to six months behind her peers at the same time as she has to cope with existent emotional insecurity. This certainly is no easy task. For many girls, it may spell the difference between success and failure.

One further area of difficulty for pregnant teen-agers should be mentioned. This concerns the attitudes of school officials. As has been mentioned, the pregnant school girl is excluded from school for periods varying from a few months to one and one-half years depending upon various circumstances, including her plans for possible surrender of the unborn infant. She may have had prior difficulty with school achievement and adjustment, and may have had an undesirable reputation within her school. If she is an inner-city student, her past educational performance may even have been poor, and the school system to which she will return will be overcrowded, with inadequate facilities and lack of individual attention. But still another factor of considerable importance arises. Not uncommonly, teen-agers, who have been pregnant, have considerable concern about the attitudes which teachers, counselors, and principals will have toward them in the future. Concerns often voiced express anxiety over being adjudged delinquent, immoral, or promiscuous. Unfortunately, there appears to be considerable truth to this fear. Principals and teachers alike, when there is knowledge of a prior pregnancy, may treat the girl as one who cannot be trusted under any circumstances. In the present author's experience, girls have not only been indirectly treated callously, with veiled aspersions, but even more direct comments have been made. School nurses have requested that girls report to their office several times weekly and have repeatedly questioned them about the possibility of repeat pregnancy. Teachers and principals have informed girls that their behavior will be watched carefully. Again, an instance can be seen where pregnancy is regarded not as being inappropriate, but as being a crime which must never be repeated. Obviously, if progress is to be made which will allow prengant teen-agers to see themselves as human beings, who have not committed a crime, but who have potentialities of leading full, meaningful, and productive lives, many changes of both a legal and attitudinal nature must be made within the educational systems throughout the country.

Y-MED EDUCATIONAL RESULTS

In light of the extremely poor educational prognosis for the pregnant teen-ager, especially the poor and/or nonwhite pregnant teen-ager, it seems appropriate to briefly look at the early educational results of the Y-MED program (Braen, 1968; Osofsky, 1967a, 1968a, 1968b). As has already been indicated, because the program has been available to all girls within the community who have been desirous of its services, because it has served primarily as a nonresidential center where few of the students have attempted concealment of the pregnancy, and because there has been a policy of exclusion of no girl, regardless of the complexity of her problems, the girls who have entered the Y-MED program have often been those with extremely complex educational difficulties. Early statistics have indicated that almost 90 percent of the girls have been operating below grade level prior to entering the program. Over 50 percent have had attendance problems prior to entering Y-MED, and almost 25 percent have had difficulties with school authorities.

The grade levels of the girls have ranged from seven to twelve. As would be anticipated, both because of previous motivational and attendance problems and because of previous experience by the majority of girls in inner-city schools, most of the girls have been behind grade level in their actual achievement. Not infrequently, individuals have entered the program two to three years behind their stated grade level. Some of the girls, in spite of having passed nine to ten grades within the school system, have been deficient in basic skills and have barely been able to read, or to write a legible sentence.

The problems of the educator have been further complicated by the variability within the group. Although many of the girls have had low I.Q. scores (again as would be anticipated because of the biases related to socioeconomic class and prior inner-city education) and prior school difficulty, a considerable number of the girls have been average or even above average educational achievers showing desire for future education. Several of the other programs for pregnant teen-agers already in existence have coped with these problems by either eliminating the low achiever, focusing primarily on the high achiever, or else by having an extremely limited educational facility. Within Y-MED, such a concept has been untenable. The feeling educationally has been that each girls should obtain the maximum education of which she is capable. Further, in addition to offering academic opportunities, schools do represent an avenue for transmitting society's standards to the student (Parsons, 1959). Therefore, the success of an educational program must also be judged by its ability to help the girls become useful and productive citizens within the society.

Although the school building used by the Y-MED program is old and no longer utilized as part of the regular school system, some very modern methods of education are in use. Insofar as the physical plant allows, team teaching and individualized instruction are used. This means that when a girl enters the program, not only are her medical, sociological, and psychological needs examined and programmed, her educational level is tested in a variety of subjects. The team of teachers decides where she is in every subject, and she then progresses at her own level. In a typical city school, with few exceptions, one must be at the same level in, for example, mathematics and English, although of course persons typically do not progress at the same level in all academic areas.

In the Y-MED school each academic subject is broken down into units, so that the girl can not only be at a different level for various academic subjects, her rate can increase at a different pace in one subject than in another. One teacher has no assigned class, thereby giving him the flexibility to tutor students. Typically, the tutorial group consists of one to four students; it should be pointed out that such individualized instruction is typically available only in the most progressive and affluent communities in this country today, although it is being provided here within the relatively low operating costs of the program.

The problems involved in operating a program incorporating such flexibility for girls with varied background, prior achievement, and present anticipations, have been complex and at times almost overwhelming. Much sensitivity has been required by the educational staff toward individual needs. Goals have had to vary, including assisting girls to function within a classroom situation, helping some indivduals to achieve meaningful saleable skills, and yet working with still others toward completion of academic programs, including preparation for college.

The results at the present time appear to be most encouraging. As must be expected in a program which caters to varied and high-risk students, not all of the girls have responded equally well to the educational program. However, the overwhelming majority of the girls have appeared to function at a much higher and more meaningful level than could have been anticipated on the basis of prior performance, school ratings, and expectations held for their socioeconomic group. During their stays within the program, the majority of girls have achieved much more educational success than could have been expected on the basis of time alone.

An early survey of the girls who have returned to regular high school programs three to twelve months following delivery, has indicated that 90 percent are still attending school. In addition, in 1967, nine girls completed requirements for their high school diplomas while attending Y-MED; a graduation was held at their request at the program facilities. (It is estimated that no more than one or two of these girls would have graduated without the program.) In 1968, present data indicates that twenty-four girls will graduate high school because of the program. It is estimated that ten, or 42 percent, of these girls will go on for post high school education—university, community college, or business school.

TABLE XIV

Y-MED EDUCATIONAL RESULTS—1968

Proportion of Girls Who Reentered Other Schools and Are Continuing to Function Successfully	90%
Estimated Number of Girls Graduating High School for Year	24
Post-High School Educational Plans:	
Business School	6
Community College	2
University	2

In addition to the obvious excitement which arises from this accomplishment, there are other implications of considerable importance. It has been estimated that in the city of Syracuse in 1967, 6,001 Negro students attended public schools. The proportions of Negro students in school declined as the age and grade level of the student increased. Twenty-two percent of elementary school pupils were Negro; 18.7 percent of junior high school students were Negro; and 11.4 percent of senior high students were Negro. Only 112 of 1,603, or 7 percent, of high school graduates were Negro. In 1968, the number of Negro high school graduates will increase slightly, but the numbers obviously will still be incredibly low. It can be expected that Y-MED will account for approximately 10 percent of these graduates in 1968.

TABLE XV

NEGRO STUDENTS BY NUMBERS AND AS A PERCENTAGE OF THE
TOTAL FOR THE SYRACUSE SCHOOL SYSTEM DURING 1967

Grade Level	*Total Enrollment*	*Negro Enrollment*	*Percent Negro*
Elementary Schools	19,166	4,207	22
Junior High Schools	5,757	1,075	18.7
Senior High Schools	5,898	675	11.4
Graduating High School Seniors	1,638	112	6.8

Personal Communication (1968)

If one program, working with some of the educationally high-est risk individuals, can so meaningfully assist individuals to achieve a higher degree of their innate potential, one is forced to ask why more high-risk students of various types are not being aided nationally. Although the author is convinced that pregnant school girls should not be involuntarily excluded from regular schools in the first place, the findings of a program, which has been designed to offer services to an otherwise unreached, forgotten, and criticized group of individuals, demonstrate that many of their problems can be solved. It is impossible to believe that the problems are not solvable for similar high-risk students in other areas, students who are at risk for a variety of reasons, of which pregnancy is only one. It is also impossible to believe that the community at large, as well as the individuals concerned, would not benefit from such attempts. Obviously, many steps need to be taken if these "unreachables" are to be reached.

V

SEX EDUCATION AND CONTRACEPTION

In this book we have examined the problems which the pregnant teen-ager faces: the inadequacies of medical, social service, and educational facilities available to her. One of the most fundamental problems of the pregnant teen-ager, however, is less vague: the right to control her own body is being denied her each day. This chapter will deal with the real problems pertaining to sex education and contraception.

Central to any discussion of teen-age mothers is a discussion of sex education and contraception. Sex education within the school systems has traditionally been denied because of puritanical ideas and notions concering its effects upon the behavior of the young (Johnson, 1966; Kirkendall, 1967). With contraception, additional problems have arisen which are related to socioeconomic class, and to the rights and responsibilities of females in general. One encouraging sign to the author is that sex education is now finally starting to be taught in the school systems of this country (American School Health Association, 1967; Johnson, 1966; Kirkendall, 1967; Luckey, 1967; SIECUS, 1965). Already many schools have begun or are considering beginning a sex education program; curriculum materials services report that the request for materials on sex education by schools, churches, community agencies, and youth organizations is great despite the relative paucity of available materials (Berry, 1967; Calderone, 1966a, b, 1967; ERIE, 1968; Fulton, 1967).

There are those who claim that sex education is adequate in its present form. They anticipate that teen-agers of both sexes have considerable knowledge about their bodies. Since studies have shown that only one-quarter of the teen-agers have received significant sex information from their parents, obviously such claims must rest upon the assumption that the education which children and teen-agers receive from peers and the mass media is adequate for their development (Peterson, 1956).

Certainly individuals' knowledge of their own sexual function is much greater today than it was a generation ago. The first menstrual period is not totally unexpected for most adolescent females, and erection and seminal emission are not unexpected by teen-age males. With the "sexual revolution" of the last twenty years, there is a general feeling that teen-agers experience less guilt about masturbation, and that both males and females have more knowledge concerning sexual function.

Yet there still remain a great deal of sexual misinformation among many teen-agers. This is especially so in areas concerning reproduction in general and, in specific, in areas relating to how pregnancy takes place and what the methods are for avoiding conception. (Unfortunately, these misconceptions are not exclusively held by the young. One is always amazed to hear the "facts," as they are expressed by some members of the adult population.)

Many teen-agers are markedly ignorant about the reproductive function of their bodies. In seminars where attendance is limited to teen-age girls, one finds boys peering through the cracks of the door trying to indirectly gain information about themselves. Not uncommonly teen-agers of both sexes, who have claimed to have accurate understanding of their bodies, have stated information which, if utilized, would be almost guaranteed to result in pregnancy unless one or both of the sexual partners was sterile. Some teen-agers report that the only safe period is midway between the menstrual periods, with the time around the period being important for abstinence. It has also been reported that if a couple has intercourse once with contraception and then again has intercourse, no contraception need be used the second time. Forms of contraception, which have been utilized and thought to be safe, have included such popular, but ineffective, items as Saran Wrap condoms and Pepsi Cola douches. One could go on and on reciting the misinformation held by teen-agers.

SEX EDUCATION: REASONS FOR NEGLECTING IT

One must logically ask, therefore, why any resistance has existed toward giving meaningful sex education to students. The answer of course is obvious, perhaps too obvious for most readers. Adults, more than the teen-agers of today, are still somewhat anxious about discussing sexual issues. Puritanical attitudes of a generation ago concerning sex have carried over into present-day adult patterns. Although adults intellectually may have freed themselves of some of the misconceptions of the past, emotionally it is difficult to unshackle oneself from traditions which have been a part of one's life. Many parents still report difficulties in discussing sex with teen-agers. Certainly, when one observes red-faced and embarrassed teachers attempting to use sexual terminology with pubescent teen-agers, one is aware, not only of the difficulty of the teen-ager, but of the difficulty of the adult. From the direct and the indirect signals from adults, teen-agers soon learn which questions are inappropriate.

Thus, very often, teen-agers are left to their own devices to find the answers to questions which may be very troublesome. Problems about biology, emotions, and attitudes perplex them, but there may be no appropriate adult to whom the teen-ager can turn.

Another issue, besides embarrassment, hinders community acceptance of sex education in the schools. Parents and educators not infrequently feel that if sex education is too open, sexual activity among teen-agers will also become more open. An unspoken, or spoken, fear concerns the possible uses to which this sexual knowledge will be put. There seems to be an assumption that if teen-agers more freely discuss sex and reproduction, even more of them will participate in premarital sexual intercourse. It is felt that freer discussions will lead to peer pressures which will result in otherwise avoidable intercourse. Somehow more open discussion of sexual issues is equated as being tantamount to adult approval of teen-age sexual promiscuity.

SOME IGNORED FACTORS

It is important to mention that such fears are not scientifically grounded (Calderone, 1965; Hayman, 1964; Kirkendall, 1967;

Peterson, 1956; WHO, 1965). No studies have found greater sexual activity among students after sex and family education courses than before the students' participation in these courses. We really do not know if sex education has any effect upon the incidence of sexual activity, but, in isolation, it seems unlikely that sex education would lead to increased activity.

Intercourse is the result of many factors: complex human emotions, the pleasure principle, physiology, social mores, and peer pressures. Sex education courses certainly would rank low on this list of factors—if such courses appeared on the list at all. Obviously, as is well known, a considerable and probably growing number of teen-agers have experienced intercourse—such experience preceding the introduction of sex education courses into the school systems. The author is convinced that teen-agers should have knowledge concerning the function of their bodies, and further, that they should have information which will assist in making the most sensible decisions involving their behavior.

One may regard sex education as what it actually is: knowledge about one's body. As in other aspects of life, if one is to use one's body properly, one is entitled to have full and rational comprehension concerning its function. If one is to accept the concept that man is a rational and thinking human being, capable of and entitled to self-control, then sex education, like other areas of knowledge, should be part of the school curriculum.

CONTRACEPTION: A MORE TOUCHY PROBLEM

The issue of contraception is a more troublesome one with which to cope. The reasons for this difficulty concern the fact that contraception must necessarily be linked to sexual activity. As with sex education, we do not know if increased contraception availability will effect the incidence of sexual activity. To condone contraceptive availability for teen-agers is not to condone sex activity and intercourse. It is an action which defines neither moral position nor obvious consequences.

The author's views concerning free love and promiscuity are irrelevant to the present book. What is important is the thesis that persons are entitled to be in control of themselves.

To the author, it seems less necessary to defend why one offers contraception to individuals than to defend why one would not offer contraception to any individual desirous of it. It is much more rational to help any female (and especially one who is single and of teen-age) to prevent an unwanted pregnancy than it is to punish her by forcing her to become pregnant against her will. And is it not, indeed, a desire to punish which makes us deny contraceptive help to one in need of it?

A PLEA FOR CONTRACEPTIVE AVAILABILITY

The plea for greater contraceptive availability for teen-agers is ultimately based upon two relevant factors. The first is that teen-agers as individuals should have the right to make decisions concerning the use of their own bodies. Each individual, as a matter of privacy and self-determination, should have this right. All evidence points to the capacity and ability of teen-agers for such decision-making (Bealer, 1964; Blos, 1962; Brittain, 1963; Halleck, 1967; Kluckholm, 1958; Lipset, 1960; Ostlund, 1957; Remmers, 1957; Rose, 1956).

The second justification for increasing contraceptive availability rests upon a reality: for a considerable number of teen-agers, pre-marital intercourse does take place. The figures may not be as high as claimed in the press, but certainly a substantial number of teen-agers, by anyone's estimate, engage in intercourse (Ehrmann, 1959; Freedman, 1965; Grinder, 1966; Halleck, 1967; Kinsey, 1948, 1953). If persons are to have intercourse, regardless of age, they are entitled to appropriate contraception. Intercourse under some circumstances may be inappropriate; society should not under any circumstances punish the participants by forcing the woman to conceive an undesired pregnancy.

The present regulations are punitive to teen-agers in general, and to teen-age girls in specific. With the exception of vaginal foam, which is relatively unknown, (and which may be markedly inconvenient for some single women), effective birth control for women can be obtained only with a prescription. Such prescriptions require a visit to a doctor. The single female under the age of twenty-one is especially disadvantaged in such a situation. If the state in which she lives rules her a minor, she must obtain parental consent to visit a physician for help, unless he is willing to violate legal statute. For many females, this makes contraception a realistic impossibility. Even if she is having intercourse, it may be difficult or even impossible for a girl to ask her mother for consent to get contraceptive help. One might argue that it would be good for a young girl to be forced into discussing this issue with her mother—possibly to be "talked out of" having intercourse. However, in addition to the burden which this places upon the mother, it is an unreality. Most girls cannot, or will not, discuss their sexual behavior with their mothers. As a result, such regulations do not result either in more frequent parent-child discussions or in a lowered incidence of intercourse; they only result in a lesser utilization of contraception.

In present day society, teen-age boys are encouraged to have intercourse, even though subtle pressures discourage their obtaining contraceptives. Yet, obviously, if conception follows intercourse, it is the girl who gets pregnant. One seldom hears a breath of criticism leveled at the selling of condoms to males over-the-counter, and without prescription. In most areas, boys at least are able to purchase condoms if their own embarrassment and if social pressures placed upon them do not make such a purchase difficult. For girls, present day rules are more restrictive. Girls do not have similar rights to contraceptive availability. To the author, this is not only discriminatory; it is senseless.

DISCRIMINATION TOWARD THE POOR

As has repeatedly been true in other areas concerning teen-age pregnancy, the issue of contraceptive availability is again compounded by poverty. In many areas a poor, and especially a young or unwed woman, faces a more complete denial of appropriate contraception than do her more affluent peers. Options of selecting physicians are not readily available to the poor, and many clinics will not dispense contraceptive prescriptions, especially if a woman is unmarried or less than a specified age.

Welfare departments, which raise so many economic questions concerning illegitimacy, contribute to the poor's difficulty in obtaining contraceptive assistance. Often, approval by a welfare commissioner is required before any *nonessential* prescription can be filled. In the case of contraception prescription, one or more months may pass before the prescription is approved. How many middle income individuals would be forced to delay obtaining contraception for several weeks? Yet, for the poor, the very society which berates illegitimacy fosters such practices.

In New York State, at the present time, Medicaid legislation exists which allows for medical care for low income individuals. Under the law, poor persons are allowed traditionally middle-class care. Yet the author has found in his community that almost all pharmacists, under apparent order from the Welfare Department, fill birth control prescriptions for only one month at a time. The rationale given relates to both the relatively slow reimbursement by the government for such prescriptions, and to the misuse of medication by a few recipients—including the sale of freely obtained pills. Whatever the reasons, such decisions result in inequality of services. The poor must report to the pharmacist once a month in contradistinction to middle-class patients who may receive supplies of pills which last three or more months. In some cases, pharmacists have denied pills to a woman when hers have been exhausted toward the end of a thirty-one day month, and have insisted that she wait until the beginning of the following month to get more pills.

For a teen-age girl, the problem is especially pertinent. She is no less embarrassed than the teen-age boy to walk into a drug store and request birth control medication from a pharmacist. Often the prescription is filled, accompained by a lecture from the pharmacist. If not, she at least suffers her own apprehensions concerning his attitudes toward her. When such difficulties are compounded by having to undergo the experience each month, the chances of not effectively utilizing contraception are increased. When further difficulties are created, such as when pharmacists refuse to fill a prescription before the beginning of a new month, the difficulties are still further compounded. In the author's experience, pregnancies have indeed resulted because of this difficulty in obtaining contraception.

THE BILL PAID BY SOCIETY AND THE INDIVIDUAL

In addition to the social pressures and stigmata placed upon the single female who becomes pregnant out of wedlock, very real legal and economic problems are raised. These problems have assumed such major consequences that legislation has been offered attempting to limit financial assistance available to women who are pregnant out of wedlock, and who are neither working nor limiting the number of their out-of-wedlock pregnancies.

The financial burden to society of out-of-wedlock pregnancies in general, and of out-of-wedlock pregnancies among teen-agers, in particular, is considerable. Sarrel (1966; 1967) at Yale, has reviewed the records of 132 girls who were pregnant at age fifteen or younger, and obtained a follow-up on each of these girls for a period of five years. The study, as others previously reported, reflects the bias of a community-oriented survey, in which middle- and upper-class girls tend to be excluded. However, because of its bias, it may be particularly pertinent in that it focuses upon girls who are likely to need community financial assistance.

The figures concerning this group of girls are quite striking. In the five years following conception of the first infant, the girls delivered an average of 3.4 additional infants, almost all of whom were delivered out of wedlock. Ninety-five percent of the girls in the study conceived at least one more child during this period of time. Of the remainder, three percent were infertile because of pelvic infection; one girl was effectively infertile because of commital to a mental institution. Ninety percent of the girls were receiving welfare assistance. In Sarrel's group, only one of the girls had received contraceptive assistance.

As has been mentioned, Krantz (1965), in a recent national survey, found evidence that the typical girl who became pregnant out of wedlock in her teens might be expected to deliver nine out-of-wedlock pregnancies during her reproductive years. Again, it cannot be too strongly emphasized that this type of study has built-in biases and, as a result, can be generalized for only certain populations. However, within the populations in-

TABLE XVI

FIVE-YEAR FOLLOW UP OF 100 PREGNANT UNMARRIED
TEEN-AGE CLINIC PATIENTS IN NEW HAVEN

Children produced	340
Number of patients who repeated pregnancy	95
Patients on welfare	60
Children produced by mothers on welfare	238
Unmarried or separated	91
Abortion	9
Contraception received	3
Venereal disease	13

From Sarrel (1966)

volved, Krantz' figures indicate that the average cost to the welfare department for one-hundred teen-age girls who are pregnant out of wedlock, and who require welfare assistance in caring for their children, is $10,000,000 over the course of the girls' lifetimes. This averages $100,000 per girl. Such a figure, while astounding at first glance, certainly can be explained. In addition, it incorporates only a fraction of the cost which is to be borne by the community. It does not account for the loss to the community of the girls' earning potentials if they had not dropped out of school, but had continued schooling and become a part of the adult productive working population. It does not include special education costs for the significant percentage of children, born under such conditions, who fail to thrive developmentally within the school systems. It does not include lower productivity which can be anticipated from high-risk children conceived under such circumstances. Thus, the staggeringly high figures, quoted by Krantz, in reality represent only one part of the real financial and human losses to be borne by the community.

In light of these considerations, it is significant to note that recent studies have indicated that teen-agers who are pregnant out of wedlock, given appropriate contraceptive assistance, demonstrate a low incidence of repeated pregnancies (Braen, 1968; Osofsky, 1968 a, b; Sarrel, 1967). Of further significance, these studies have also been done with lower socioeconomic populations, where previous information had indicated that a high rate of repeated pregnancies might be anticipated. Thus, one can see that when teen-age girls are given the opportunity to control their own bodies—the opportunity to avoid pregnancy—such opportunity is very frequently utilized.

If most girls who are pregnant in their teens would voluntarily prefer to avoid future pregnancy, and if these girls use contraceptive techniques when available, cannot the conclusions be carried over to other teen-age girls who do not happen to be pregnant? The answer is obvious. It certainly would appear likely that nonpregnant teen-agers, like their pregnant peers, would prefer not to be pregnant at this time in their lives. If appropriate sex education is available, and if appropriate contraception is also made available, it is likely, bordering on certain, that many unwanted teen-age pregnancies can be avoided. The potential humanistic and developmental benefits for the teen-agers involved, the social and emotional benefits for their families, and the very real economic gains to the community and the civilization as a whole—these assets cannot even be measured, but can certainly be assumed to be large indeed.

VI

ABORTION

It has been estimated that as many as two and a half million abortions are performed each year in this country. Over half, (the figure sometimes is cited as four out of five) are performed on married women. Most are performed illegally; medical complications and even occasional maternal death result from these procedures. In the United States, abortions account for one-fifth of all maternal deaths and thus represent the largest single cause of maternal mortality. Obviously, completely accurate statistics concerning abortion incidence are impossible, because abortion is an illegal activity. However, the available data, inaccurate as it may be, clearly demonstrates that many women in this country obtain abortions annually and that significant medical problems result because of the illegality and resultant lack of safety of most of these abortions (Thompson, 1964; U.S. Dept. of Health, Education and Welfare, 1966; Williams, 1966; Roemer, 1967).

There is perhaps no more fundamental human right, save the right to life itself, than the right to one's own physical person. A basic part of this right is that of determining whether or not one will give birth to another human being. To the author, an egg, a sperm, a zygote, or even a fetus cannot yet be considered a person or a human being. Whatever rights these may have, should be because of biological fact completely dependent upon, and subordinate to, the human bodies which house them.

REVIEW OF LAWS

At the present time, one can categorically state that allowed indications for abortion in this country are considerably more restrictive than in most other areas of the world (Roemer, 1967; NOW, 1967; Tietze, 1967).

Criminal abortion laws in forty-two states prohibit the performance of abortions unless necessary to save the life of the pregnant woman. In the other eight states—Alabama, California, Colorado, Maryland, Mississippi, New Mexico, North Carolina, and Oregon—and in the District of Columbia, abortions are permitted in certain other additional circumstances, such as where pregnancy results from rape, incest, or where the physical or mental health of the woman is endangered.

Bills to make abortion laws less restrictive were introduced in twenty-eight state legislatures in 1967. The Colorado and North Carolina laws, enacted in 1967, are patterned after the American Law Institute's Model Penal Code. They permit abortions where continuance of the pregnancy would gravely impair the physical or mental health of the woman; the child would be born with grave physical or mental defect; or the pregnancy resulted from rape, incest or other felonious intercourse. (It may be noted that the definition of *human being* in the ALI Penal Code criminal homicide provisions is *a person who has been born and is alive.*)

In the majority of states, infant and social problems are not mentioned as possible indications for therapeutic abortion. Genetic traits which predictably result in fetal malformations, induction of drugs which lead to anomalies, and such diseases as German Measles, even when occurring at six weeks of gestation when severe anomalies can be anticipated in 50 percent of the cases, are not legal indications for abortion.

It, therefore, is obvious that attitudes and laws in the United States are quite dissimilar from those existing in other countries (Roemer, 1967; Tietze, 1967; Field, 1956; Mehlah, 1966; Borell, 1966). Since the 1930's, the Scandinavian countries have authorized abortions for socio-medical or "extended medical reasons." Physician approval is required, but the indications include a wide variety of socially-oriented indications. Japanese legislation has, since 1948, allowed abortions to be performed for social, as well as medical, indications. Abortion is, in effect, available to almost all Japanese women. The Soviet Union, Hungary, and Bulgaria, in order to decrease harm to the health of women from abortions performed outside of hospitals, have gone a step further in recognizing the rights of women. In the 1950's these countries enacted legislation which provides for abortion upon the demand of the individual woman. A physician may discuss any relevant social and medical facts, but abortion can be denied only if there are medical contradictions.

A SOCIO-HISTORICAL PERSPECTIVE

Abortion is the oldest known procedure in the history of gynecology. Abortion was practiced in every major civilization, although some of the techniques utilized might seem barbaric by present day standards. One could go through the development of philosophies which have allowed ethnic, religious, and national groups to either accept or reject abortion, but such a discussion appears inappropriate for the scope of this book. What can be stated is that historically a wide variety of interpretations were made depending upon the culture and attitude of the groups involved.

In some societies abortion is not only condoned, but encouraged. In Japan, for example, although contraception is now encouraged to diminish the incidence of abortion, abortion serves as a method of birth control to halt population growth and is, perhaps, still more popular for this function than contraception (Roemer, 1967). The opposite extreme can be seen in the view of the Catholic church, which defines abortion as a sin because of the termination of fetal life. Of some note, prior to 1869, the Catholic church's attitude was considerably different. The small fetus was defined as not having a soul; aborting it, therefore, did not destroy a life. Only since 1869 has the definition of life been extended backward to preclude the performance of all abortions.

In the United States, at the present time, many persons are opposed to easing or removing the legal barriers to obtaining abortions. For some, the objections are on religious grounds. Since the Catholic church forbids abortion as a primary procedure, a considerable percentage of the population has religious difficulty accepting such progressive changes in the laws. However, there are many persons, Catholic and non-Catholic alike, who oppose these changes because of individual conviction.

Abortion is not the most desirable method of birth control, and other means should be made available to everyone who wishes to use them. The ease and medical safety of contraception justify its being the primary method of birth control. With any form of abortion, no matter how aseptic the technique, there is always the risk of morbidity, and even occasional mortality, for the mother; with repeated abortions the incidence of gynecological complications, which may lead to sterility, rises slightly.

The relevant question which must be raised, however, is not whether contraception is preferable to abortion for birth control, but whether legally sanctioned abortions should be allowed for unwanted pregnancies after these pregnancies have been conceived. After conception, contraception obviously offers no answer. Unwanted pregnancies must either be carried to term or abortions must be performed.

Criminal abortion laws clearly have proven to be ineffectual in eliminating the use of abortion as a means of birth control. All that they have succeeded in accomplishing is to drive women to unskilled practitioners or to those doctors who are willing to violate the law.

THE CASE OF PROHIBITION

When prohibition against the sale of liquor in this country was enacted, moral, ethical, and philosophical arguments were used in justifying the law. However, prohibition did not succeed: liquor was sold; its price went up, with even low quality liquor costing astronomically high sums. In addition, since the manufacturing of liquor was illegal, the whole industry went underground, reaping huge profits to underworld criminals, who were, one can be certain, happy indeed to have the drinking industry given to them. The behavior of the populus toward the prohibition of liquor was dissimilar to that which existed toward other types of crime. Whereas a large segment of the population would illegally purchase liquor, a similarly large group never robbed banks or homes.

The case of prohibition in this country pointed out an important principle. Almost all human beings were able to collectively agree that many types of crime and injury toward one's neighbor were reprehensible and undesirable. Few members of society questioned calling these acts criminal, and few people questioned punishing individuals for agreed upon criminal acts. Drinking, however, was a special case. What appeared ethical and morally appropriate to one group was quite contrary to the considered evaluation and decisions of another group. The act was unenforceable; prohibition was repealed.

It is obvious that one can make a similar case for abortion. Here, too, one sees a group of legal statutes which are, in reality, unenforceable. Once again, one can see individuals within the populace who would never consider an abortion for themselves, others who would consider abortion under select circumstances, and still others who consider abortion to be a reasonable alternative to any undesired pregnancy. As opposed to the situation prevalent with most illegal activities, the police and members of the district attorney's staff rarely pursue the issue and bring the individual women into court. Physicians and hospitals are loath to give out information concerning women who have admitted obtaining criminal abortions. Most citizens would be offended if a trial were to occur in which a mother of ten were sent to jail because an eleventh pregnancy, under conditions of emotional and financial poverty, were interrupted at her doing.

THE CIVIL RIGHTS OF WOMEN

The introduction referred to the abstract discussion which so frequently is heard regarding the rights of the fetus. The question of both when life begins and when viability occurs is often raised. Although no answer which would be satisfactory to all can be given, debates ensue because of concern over the well-being of the fetus. It is ironic that little similar concern has been raised for the well-being of the already living woman who has to bear this fetus. Relatively few voices have been raised concerning the woman's rights: whether she should be forced to bear an unwanted child against her will. The question not only exists of whether one should avoid the complications of illegal abortion, including pelvic infection and death. A further question must be raised as to whether present day concepts of the dignity and rights of women do not include their having a say in whether an undesired pregnancy, for whatever social and medical indications, must be borne.

It is somewhat comforting to the author that the American Civil Liberties Union (1968) has recently decided to place itself on record by its willingness to uphold the civil right of a woman to obtain an abortion. It would seem as though modern day concepts make such an attitude and decision mandatory.

State criminal abortion laws should be repealed. A woman should have the civil right to determine, within medical limits of safety, whether or not an abortion be obtained.

One alternate and acceptable solution, proposed by the National Organization for Women (1967), is to replace, rather than repeal, the present statutes. Their suggested legislation makes it the woman's right to determine whether she should, or of equal importance, whether she should not obtain an abortion. The rationale for this proposed legislation rests upon the fear that despite the prohibition which exists at present against most abortions, future social welfare rules or legislation may require abortions under certain social circumstances—including illegitimacy and poverty. The group, therefore, feels it necessary to mention the woman's right to elect to bear a "socially undesirable" child. Either way, with repeal or with alternate legislation, the important issue is to recognize the civil rights of women.

In light of the context of the present book, it is particularly ironic to view the effects of present day legislation upon teen-agers. Even in those states where abortion laws are most liberal, no girl age sixeen or older is eligible for legal abortion with social indications. In most states, regardless of age, females are not eligible for abortion with social indications. Yet, at the same time, girls are excluded from school because of pregnancy, are given less than adequate social assistance, and often are provided with inferior medical care. Prior sex education within the schools has been notoriously non-existent. And finally, because of age, if not because of sex, the girl has been denied contraceptive protection to prevent the unwanted pregnancy. It would certainly seem as though the civil rights of the individual have long been ignored.

Perhaps, in view of the almost total lack of attention which has been paid to the civil rights of women in the area of abortion, it is worth briefly looking at the role of females in general. Throughout the ages, and in every major culture, the role of women has been submissive, passive, and docile. In many cultures, women have had no legal rights. Even their children were not their own possessions, but were rather the possessions of the husband during his lifetime, and of the husband's family following his death. Every major religious group has elevated men to a more significant position than that granted to women. The right to vote has been a relatively recent one, and even now, female representation in governing bodies is mere tokenism. Job opportunities are obviously limited; pay and promotion scales for women are far lower than they are in similar cases for men (DeBeauvoir, 1953).

In viewing abortion legislation, one can see a further link in this chain of sex role differential. The legislators, who make the decisions, and the judges, who interpret the decisions, are almost uniformly male. Speakers who debate the issue are male—clergymen, physicians, and civic leaders.

An example of this point is the International Conference on Abortion, held in Washington, D.C., September 7–9, 1967. This major conference divided the pertinent issues on abortion into legal, sociological, ethical, and medical domains. Forty-eight persons were on the panel; only three were women. One woman was a physician, the other two, academicians. Of some note, the three were among the most militant in the group which, however, generally agreed that abortion laws should be repealed.

The few women who occasionally have a say on the abortion issue are typically too old, or too rich and sophisticated, to be in the relevant group. Should middle- or upper-class women conceive an unwanted pregnancy, they can easily find a safe, if illegal and expensive, abortion. How often does one see women from the lower socioeconomic group on such panels? How often does one see a woman who has had a kitchen table abortion on such panels? How often does one see a teen-ager who has been deprived of education because of pregnancy on the panel? The answer to all of these questions is *never*.

It is unfortunate that in an era when poor blacks are finally being given at least token representation in governing and decision-making councils, rather than allowing decisions on their behalf to be made strictly by whites and middle-class blacks, that women, and especially those women who are potential candidates for abortion, either now or in the future, or who have had abortions in the past, are given little representation in decision-making groups. Those who are most intimately involved are excluded from decision-making roles; those who are in decision-making roles moralize and philosophize, but do not consider the real and meaningful problems which exist for the involved individuals. And of significance, abortions continue to occur.

Perhaps our present abortion laws suffer from cultural lag; our society functions under the premises of self-determination, individualism, and the importance of the good life for each member. However, in an instance of as basic a life issue as bearing a child, we do not yet grant this self-determination.

PUNITIVE EFFECTS OF LEGISLATION UPON THE POOR

An issue of major importance is that of the differential effect of present abortion legislation upon the poor. As we have seen, the problems of pregnant teen-agers are often those of the poor, and especially the nonwhite members of society. Previously cited figures have indicated that the overwhelming majority of illegal abortions are performed upon white women (Kinsey, 1958). Similarly, the overwhelming majority of hospital-approved therapeutic abortions are performed upon middle- and upper-class private patients (Gold, 1965). This is in spite of the statistics which indicate that sixty percent of infants delivered out of wedlock are delivered to nonwhite mothers. Since a large number of pregnancies are conceived under less than appropriate circumstances for women of all ethnic backgrounds, but since the majority of abortions are performed upon white, and undoubtedly middle-and upper-class women, one is forced to ask, why is this so? Is it possible that once again existing legislation fosters discrimination toward the poor? The answer, to the author, is : *Yes.*

While existing laws may be discriminatory to women in general, they are definitely discriminatory to women from lower socioeconomic classes, and especially, therefore, to nonwhite women. If a white, middle-class woman desires an abortion, it is possible for her to obtain one. In many areas, it is even possible for her to obtain one safely, although this is certainly not always the case. She may, on the basis of prior knowledge obtained from friends or even from physicians, be able to receive an abortion in a legally accredited hospital, or at least in a facility which is relatively medically safe.

For the poor, the situation is quite different. Preparations and techniques used to induce abortion among the poor may be quite ineffective as far as producing the desired result for the patient. In addition, as is obvious to the medical community, the types of abortions performed under such circumstances are considerably less than safe, with jeopardy of a marked nature to the woman. The abortions received by the poor and by the unknowledgeable are certainly conducive to a high incidence of crippling infection, and even death. The question may be asked as to why the poor obtain less safe abortions. Part of the difference may be due to a relative lack of medical sophistication. Knowledge concerning appropriate, effective, and safe techniques of abortion is related to educational background and to socioeconomic class.

The incidence of dangerous abortion among the poor, however, is much higher than can be accounted for by differences in medical sophistication. Mainly the differential is related to being poor —to not having several hundred dollars at one's disposal.

Therapeutic abortions performed in accredited hospitals usually require, at a minimum, the testimony of two physicians concerning the overwhelming danger of the pregnancy to the mother's health. Frequently these physicians are psychiatrists. The more affluent members of society can better afford both the consultations and the subsequent treatment. In addition, the physician evaluation is more likely to be favorable for middle- and upper-class women than it is for the poor (Gold, 1965).

Of further significance, obviously the great proportion of abortions in this country are performed for non-medical indications and are illegal. With relatively few exceptions, safe abortions, under these circumstances, are very expensive and may require the patient's journeying to another community or even to another country. For the poor, knowledge of the availability of such procedures is not always absent. But even if the knowledge is available, the poor patient is still in the bind of being unable to afford such a procedure. With a minimum of several hundred dollars being the rule rather than the exception, few poor patients can afford the cost of a medically safe abortion.

One may even ask whether the much higher incidence of live out-of-wedlock births among the poor is related to the relative paucity of safe abortions available to members of this socio-economic class. The majority of the poor are not as medically unsophisticated as would be imagined by the middle-class population, and even among those who are relatively medically unsophisticated concerning the existence of safe abortion, there is coexistent knowledge of the danger and even the ineffectiveness of the abortions available to them. Therefore, it is logical to expect economically deprived individuals to acquiesce to carrying an unwanted pregnancy.

Thus, again, one sees an all too familiar condition. Just as the poor and the nonwhite receive lower quality medical care, inadequate social service, fewer educational opportunities, and less chance in general to determine their own fates, they are also disadvantaged in the area of abortion.

The poor are criticized for their number of illegitimate pregnancies. Yet for them, effective contraception is less available. Effective and safe abortion, by middle-class standards, is almost nonexistent. For the middle and upper classes, the present abortion laws may be unfair and unrealistic. For the lower socio-economic groups, the present laws are clearly discriminatory.

CONCLUDING NOTES

This book has taken a look at some of the problems which confront pregnant teen-agers. To identify and scrutinize these problems is a difficult task. Studies, reports, and statistics dealing with pregnancy in this young age group are often biased severely. Data collection tends to protect the white and more affluent members of society. Even honestly attempted experiments are plagued by both internal and external biases.

However, in spite of these limitations, it has become obvious that pregnant teen-agers are indeed at risk and that they do face many difficulties. It has also been seen over and over again that these difficulties are compounded by factors related to poverty, race, illegitimacy, age, and female gender.

Medically, the pregnant teen-ager is clearly in jeopardy. Serious complications are more often present in this group than they are among pregnant women at large. Both prematurity and perinatal mortality are extremely prevalent. The surviving infants are plagued by a much higher incidence of developmental and neurological complications. Yet little meaningful effort is made by the medical community to prevent and control these problems. Long waits in impersonal and crowded clinics are the rule rather than the exception. Socially acceptable middle- and upper-class patients receive the most adequate and dedicated care; yet these are the patients who would do relatively well under any adequate circumstances. Patients, who because of intertwined medical and social reasons, are at highest risk, receive disproportionately little interest and attention. Results of programs, which have provided both empathy and fine quality of care, have dispelled the myth which has long suggested that such patients are *unreachable*. These patients *can* be helped if a meaningful effort is made.

When one looks at the figures concerning social service counseling, the conclusion emerges that in this area things are, if anything, worse. Because of the financial cost to the community resulting from out-of-wedlock pregnancies, the average lay and professional person believes that an abundance of counseling exists. Maternity homes for individuals pregnant out of wedlock are assumed to meet many of the problems. Yet the facts again give information quite to the contrary. Maternity homes give services to but a small percentage of women; by virtue of their criteria, they cater to the white and somewhat affluent women. Other services provided by communities, voluntary agencies, and hospitals are sparse indeed. Where existent, they, too, cater to white, middle- and upper-class individuals. Effective services for the poor, and especially for the nonwhite, are almost nonexistent. Adoption may not be presented as a meaningful option. The prospective mothers are encouraged to quit school and abandon plans for future meaningful employment. Positive counseling may consist only of assisting the individuals to make application for welfare funds.

The educational situation confronting pregnant teen-agers is also discouraging. Here, punitive societal attitudes towards pregnant girls interact disadvantageously with problems resultant from race, prejudice, and poverty. Schools do not create all of society's problems—but here they certainly contribute. The educational system represents a meaningful avenue for enculturating all Americans into the socially acceptable middle class; as in other areas, this responsibility is abdicated when it pertains to pregnant teen-agers. Options are unavailable to pregnant school girls. They are excluded from school summarily; in some cases permanent exclusion is mandatory. For the poor and nonwhite, who are often keeping their infants, the situation is even more prejudicial than it is for the middle and upper classes. Their prior educational experience has been in slum schools. As a result, their school level of achievement at the time they become pregnant is already far behind that set for peers in more favored economic areas. Yet, whereas the more affluent may miss a few to several months of school and may, because of falsified records, be able to reenter without the stigma of being pregnant out of wedlock, the poor are frequently excluded for up to one and one-half years. When this long exclusion is further compounded by a history of underachievement and lack of interest; when welfare workers typically counsel these individuals not to return to school; and when the return, if at all, is to take place in a less than adequate slum school, where discipline rather than education may represent the primary effort; it is not surprising that follow-up results are poor. Relatively few of the economically poor pregnant females return to school. Of those who do, the success rate is low. Again, it has been shown that a meaningful effort can reverse this wasteful trend.

When one looks at the issues involved with sex education, contraception, and abortion policies, similar by discouraging data is uncovered. Puritanical notions have prevented adequate sex education in this country. Yet it is often assumed that all teen-agers are knowledgeable about the functioning of their bodies— an unwarranted assumption. Relatively few teen-agers have had meaningful instruction from parents and appropriate adult authorities. For some, at least, an unwanted pregnancy represents an honest mistake concerning reproductive facts. With contraception, similar problems exist. Males are tacitly, and in some cases, directly encouraged to have intercourse; they can freely purchase contraception if they are not too embarrassed to do so. Adolescent females, who become pregnant and bear the babies, are, however, denied contraception. Most forms of contraception are available to them only with a physician's prescription; physicians cannot be seen without parental consent. If an unwanted conception takes place, external societal problems continue for the female. The very society which both criticizes the adolescent for her supposed promiscuity and at the same time denies her contraception to prevent pregnancy complains about the financial burden to the community. This same society does not allow her the civil right of fully being able to control her own body— to obtain an abortion. The unwanted fetus is protected; the living female is ignored.

As the book has demonstrated, the cost of this punitive medical, educational, and social behavior is high indeed. The financial burden has been almost staggering; it has received much public and legislative concern. What has unfortunately received less concern is the social and human wastage—wastage which further contributes to the mounting financial community cost: the girls do not complete their education; meaningful jobs are closed to them; they stay home and raise one or more infants— often under circumstances of developmental jeopardy; they are indirectly pushed onto welfare rolls.

What irony it is that a society which denies sex education, contraception, and abortion, a society which gives less than adequate medical care and almost nonexistent counseling, and a society which unilaterally excludes educationally high-risk girls from school because of the noncriminal condition of pregnancy, is the same society which publicly condemns the female who is pregnant out of wedlock.

There is a homily which states that one can tell if a person means what he says if he *puts his money where his mouth is.* Our society claims to be humanistic and moralistic. It claims to be interested in individuals—especially the youth of the nation. Yet these prejudicial conditions exist. Appropriate options and opportunities are unavailable for a large group of human beings. Are we—is our society—truly willing to make the commitment which is claimed to exist? Are we willing to deal with these unanswered problems? With meaningful effort they *can be* solved.

REFERENCES

ACLU Backs Right to Abortion: Civil Liberties, January 1968, p. 3.

ADAMS, H. M., and GALLAGHER, V. M.: Some facts and observations about illegitimacy. *Children, 10:*43, 1963.

ANDERSON, E. W.; HAMILTON, M. W., and KENNA, J. C.: Psychiatric, social and psychological aspects of illegitimate pregnancy in girls under sixteen years. *Psychiat Neurol (Basel), 133:*207, 1957.

American Hospital Association: *Hospital Statistics, 1961.* Hospitals, August 1, 1962, Part 2, Chart 2, p. 404.

ARMIJO, R., and MONREAL, T.: El problema del aborto provacado en Chile. *Bol Ofic sanit panamer, 60(1):*39, 1966.

AZNAR, R., and BENNETT, A. E.: Pregnancy in the adolescent girl. *Amer J Obstet Gynec, 81:*934, 1961.

BATTAGLIA, F. C.; FRAZIER, T. M., and HELLEGERS, A. E.: Obstetric and pediatric complications of juvenile pregnancy. *Pediatrics, 32:* 902, 1963.

BATTAGLIA, F. C.; FRAZIER, T. M., and HELLEGERS, A. E.: Birth weight, gestational age, and pregnancy outcome, with special reference to high birth weight—low gestational age infant. *Pediatrics, 37:* 417, 1966.

BEALER, R. C.; WILLITS, F. K., and MAIDA, P. R.: The rebellious youth subculture—a myth. *Children, 11:*43, 1964.

BELL, R.: The One-Parent Mother in the Negro Lower Class. p. 9, (unpublished paper).

BENEDICT, R.: Continuities and discontinuities in cultural conditioning. In Mead, M. and Wolfenstein, M. (Eds.): *Childhood in Contemporary Cultures.* Chicago, U. of Chicago, 1955, pp. 21–30.

Berean Institute: A Positive Approach to Unmarried Mothers. First and second progress reports. Philadelphia, Pa., November 1959 to November 1960.

BERESFORD, J. C., and RIVLIN, A. M.: The Multigeneration Family. Presented at University of Michigan Conference on Aging, Ann Arbor, July 1964, p. 11 and Appendix Table 1, (unpublished paper).

BERL, M. E.: An interim school program for unwed mothers. *Child Welfare, 39:*22, January, 1960.

BERNARD, J.: *American Family Behavior.* New York, Harper, 1942, p. 522.

BERNARD, J.: *Marriage and Family Among Negroes.* New Jersey, Prentice-Hall, 1966.

BERNSTEIN, B., and SAUBER, M.: *Deterrents to Early Prenatal Care and Social Services Among Women Pregnant Out-of-Wedlock.* Albany, New York State Department of Social Welfare, 1960, 179 pp. (Study made by the Community Council of Greater New York.)

BERNSTEIN, R.: Are we still stereotyping the unmarried mother? *Social Work,* 5:22, 1960.

BERNSTEIN, R.: Gaps in services to unmarried mothers. *Children, 10:* 49, 1963.

BERRY, G. P.: The SIECUS purpose. SIECUS 1967—Retrospect and Prospect. *SIECUS Newsletter,* Vol. 2, No. 4, New York, Winter 1967.

BETTELHEIM, B.: The problem of generations. In Erikson, E. H. (Ed.): *Youth: Change and Challenge.* New York, Basic Books, 1963, pp. 63–92.

BILLINGSLEY, A., and BILLINGSLEY, A. T.: Illegitimacy and patterns of Negro family life. In Roberts, R. W. (Ed.): *The Unwed Mother.* New York, Harper, 1966, p. 133.

BINGHAN, A. T.: Determinants of sex delinquency in adolescent girls— based on intensive studies of 500 cases. *J Amer Inst Crim Law Criminology, 13:*494, 1922–23.

BIRCH, H. G.: Health and Education of Socially Disadvantaged Children. Presented at conference on Bio-Social Factors in the Development and Learning of Disadvantaged Children held in Syracuse, April, 1967.

BLEIBERG, N.; JACOBZINER, H.; RICH, H., and MERCHANT, R.: Young unmarried mothers in child health stations of two New York City districts. *Amer J Public Health, 52(12):*2030, 1962.

BLOCK, B.: The unmarried mother—Is she different? *The Family, 26:* 163, 1945.

BLOOM, S. W.: *The Doctor and His Patient.* New York, Free Press, 1963.

BOEHM, W. W.: Sociocultural factors in adolescent unmarried motherhood. *Casework Papers,* 1960–61, pp. 93–107.

BLOS, PETER: *On Adolescence: A Psychoanalytic Interpretation.* New York, Free Press, 1962.

BONAN, A. F.: Psychoanalytic implications in treating unmarried mothers with narcissistic character structures. *Social Casework,* 44:323, 1963.

BORELL, U., and ENGSTROM, L.: Legal abortions in Sweden. *World Med J*, *13*:72, 1966.

BOWMAN, L. A.: The unmarried mother who is a minor. *Child Welfare*, *37*:13, October 1958.

BRAEN, B. B.; DIFLORIO, R.; HAGEN. J. H.; LONG, R.; OSOFSKY, H. J., and WOOD, P. M.: A Multi-Disciplinary Program for Unwed Pregnant Adolescents—A Progress Report. Presented at the American Orthopsychiatric Convention in Chicago, March 1968.

BRITTAIN, C. V.: Adolescent choices and parent-peer cross-pressures. *Amer Sociol Rev*, *28*:385 June 1963.

BROWN, R.: *Social Psychology*. New York, Free Press, 1965.

BURCHINAL, L.: School policies and school age marriages. *J Family Life Ed*, March 1960.

BURKHEAD, J.: *Input and Output in Large City Schools*. Syracuse, Syracuse, 1967.

CALDERONE, M. S.: Sex and the teen-ager—and the physician. *The Year Book of Obstetrics and Gynecology*. 1965–1966, pp. 284–293.

CALDERONE, M. S.: Sex and the adolescent. *Clin Pediat*, *5*:171, 1966.

CALDERONE, M. S.: Sex education in medical education. *Marquette Med Rev*, *32(3)*:64. Summer Issue, 1966.

CALDERONE, M. S.: Community responsibility for sex education. *SIECUS Newsletter* (*New York*) Vol. 3, No. 1, Spring, 1967.

CAMPBELL, D. T., and STANLEY, J. C.: Experimental and quasi-experimental designs for research on teaching. In Gage, N. L. (Ed.): *Handbook of Research on Teaching*. Chicago, Rand McNally, 1963, pp. 171–246.

CHILDERS, A. T.: Some notes on sex mores among Negro children. *Amer J Orthopsychiat*, *6*:442, 1936.

CHILMAN, C.: Child-rearing and family relationship patterns of the very poor. *Welfare in Rev*, January 1965, p. 9.

CHRISTENSEN, H. T.: Scandinavian and American sex norms: Some comparisons with sociological implications. *J Soc Issues*, *22*:60, 1966.

COLEMAN, J. S.: *Equality of Educational Opportunity*. U.S. Government Printing Office. Washington, 1966.

DAY, G. A.: A program for teen-age unwed mothers. *Amer J Public Health*, *55*:978, 1965.

DEBEAUVOIR, S.: *The Second Sex*. New York, Knopf, 1953.

DERTHICK, L. C.: Elimination of Roadblocks in Education of School-Age Unmarried Mothers. Paper presented at annual meeting at Florence Crittenden Homes, Atlantic City, N. J., 1960.

DEUTSCH, H.: *The Psychology of Women: A Psychoanalytic Inter-pretation.* New York, Grune, 1945, Vol. II, Chap. X.

DEUTSCH, M., *et al.: The Disadvantaged Child.* New York, Basic Books, 1967.

DIBBLE, M. V.; BRIN, M.; MCMULLEN, E.; PEEL, A., and CHEN, N.: Some preliminary biochemical findings in junior high school children in Syracuse and Onondaga County, New York. *Amer J Clin Nutr, 17*:218, 1965.

DONABEDIAN, A.; ROSENFELD, L. S., and SOUTHERN, E. M.: Infant mortality and socioeconomic status in a metropolitan community. *Public Health Rep, 80*:1083, 1965.

DONNELL, C., and GLICK, S. J.: Background factors in 100 cases of Jewish unmarried mothers. *Jew Soc Serv Quart, 29*:152, 1952.

DRILLIEN, C. M.: A longitudinal study of the growth and development of prematurely and naturally born children. III. Mental development. *Arch Dis Child, 34*:37, 1959.

DRILLIEN, C. M.: The growth and development of the prematurely born infant. Baltimore, Williams & Wilkins, 1964.

Eastern Regional Institute for Education: Curriculum Materials Information Service, 1968. (Personal communications).

EASTMAN, N. J., and HELLMAN, L. M. (Eds.): *Williams Obstetrics,* 12th ed. New York, Appleton, 1961.

Editors of Education USA: *The Scope of Education of 1966–1967.* National School Public Relations Association, 1966, p. 64.

EDLIN, S. B.: *The Unmarried Mother in our Society.* New York, Farrar, Straus, 1954.

EHRMANN, W.: *Premarital Dating Behavior.* New York, Henry Holt, 1959.

EISENSTADT, S. N.: Archetypal patterns of youth. In Erikson, E. H. (Ed.): *Youth: Change and Challenge.* New York, Basic Books, 1963, pp. 24–42.

ERIKSON, E. H. (Ed.): *Youth: Change and Challenge.* New York, Basic Books, 1963.

ERIKSON, E. H.: Youth: fidelity and diversity. *Youth: Change and Challenge.* New York, Basic Books, 1963, pp. 1–23.

FIELD, M. G.: The re-legalization of abortion in Soviet Russia. *New Eng J Med, 255*:421, 1956.

FINE, BENJAMIN: *Underachievers.* New York, Dutton, 1967.

FOSTER, G. R.: Sex information vs. sex education: Implications for school health. *J Sch Health, 37*:248, 1967.

FOWLER, I.: The relationship of certain perinatal factors to behavior, speech, or learning problems in children. *Southern Med J, 58:* 1245, 1965.

FRAZIER, E. F.: *The Negro Family in the United States.* Chicago, U. of Chicago, 1939, Chapt. VI, p. 108.

FREEDMAN, M. B.: Some theoretical and practical implications of a longitudinal study of college women. *Psychiatry, 26:*176, 1963.

FREEDMAN, M. B.: The sexual behavior of American college women. *Merrill Palmer Quart, 11:*33, 1965.

FREUD, A.: Adolescence. In Eissler, R.S. *et al.* (Eds.): *Psychoanalytic Study of the Child.* New York, Int. Univs., *13:*255, 1958.

FREUD, A.: *The Ego and the Mechanisms of Defense.* New York, Int. Univs., 1946.

FRIEDENBERG, E. Z.: *The Vanishing Adolescent.* Boston, Beacon, 1959.

FROST, J., and HAWKES, G. R.: *The Disadvantaged Child—Issue and Innovations.* Boston, Houghton, 1966.

FULTON, W. C.: Why is there a sex information and education council of the United States? Why a new, separate organization? *J Sch Health, 37:*232, 1967.

GALLAGHER, J. R.: Adolescents: physiologic and psychologic characteristics. *Clin Pediat, 2:*151, 1963.

GEBHARD, P., *et al.: Pregnancy, Birth and Abortion.* New York: Harper, 1958.

GLICK, P. C.: Marriage instability: Variations by size of place and region, *Milbank Memorial Fund Quart, 41:*46, January, 1963.

GOLD, E. M.: A broad view of maternity care. *Children, 9:*52, 1962.

GOLD, E. M.; ERHARDT, C. L.; JACOBZINER, H., and NELSON, F. G.: Therapeutic abortions in New York City: Twenty-year review. *Amer J Public Health, 55(7):*964, 1965.

GOLD, E. M.: Observations on abortion. *World Med J, 13(3):*76, 1966.

GOLDSMITH, J. K.: The unmarried mother's search for standards. *Soc Casework, 38:*69, 1957.

GOODE, W. J.: Illegitimacy in the Caribbean social structure. *Amer Soc Rev, 25:*21, 1960.

GOODE, W. J.: Illegitimacy, anomie, and cultural penetration. *Amer Soc Rev, 26:*910, 1961.

GOODMAN, P.: *Growing Up Absurd.* New York, Vintage Books, 1956.

GOTTSCHALK, L. A.; TITCHENER, J. L.; PIKER, H. N., and STEWART, S. S.: Psycho-social factors associated with pregnancy in adolescent girls. A preliminary report. *J Ner Ment Dis, 138:*524, 1964.

GRINDER, R. E., and SCHMIDT, S. S.: Coeds and contraceptive information. *J Marriage Family,* 28:471, 1966.

GUIBORD, A. S. B., and PARKER, I. R.: *What Becomes of the Unmarried Mother?* Boston, Research Bureau on Social Casework, 1922.

HALLECK, S. L.: Sex and mental health on the campus. *JAMA, 200:* 108, 1967.

HARTER, C. L., and BEASLEY, J. D.: A survey concerning induced abortions in New Orleans. *Amer J Public Health,* 57:1937, 1967.

HARTLEY, S. M.: The amazing rise of illegitimacy in Great Britain. *Social Forces,* 44:533, 1965–1966.

HASSAN, H. M., and FALLS, F. H.: The young primipara. A clinical study. *Amer J Obstet Gynec,* 88:256, 1964.

Help for the Asking: A Study of Unwed Parents and Services to Them in Metropolitan Boston. Research Department, United Community Services of Metropolitan Boston, Jan. 1964.

HERTZ, H., and LITTLE, S. W.: Unmarried Negro mothers in a Southern urban community. *Social Forces,* 23:73, 1944.

HERZOG, E.: Some assumptions about the poor. *Social Serv Rev,* 37(4):389, 1963.

HERZOG, E., and BERNSTEIN, R.: *Health Services for Unmarried Mothers.* U.S. Department of Health, Education and Welfare, Welfare Administration, Children's Bureau, 1964.

HERZOG, E.: The chronic revolution: Births out of wedlock. *Clin Pediat,* 5:130, 1966.

HIMES, J. S.: Some reactions to a hypothetical premarital pregnancy by one hundred Negro college women. *J Marriage Family,* 26: 364, 1964.

HOLT, J.: *How Children Fail.* New York, Pitman, 1964.

HOLT, J.: *How Children Learn.* New York, Pitman, 1967.

HUTCHINSON, B.: Unmarried mothers as patients of a psychiatric clinic. *Smith College Studies in Social Work,* 19:102, 1949.

Illegitimacy—Data and Findings for Prevention, Treatment and Policy Formulation. New York, National Council on Illegitimacy, Oct. 1965.

Infant and perinatal mortality in the United States. *Vital and Health Statistics—Analytical Studies.* National Center for Health Statistics. U.S. Department of Health, Education and Welfare. Public Health Service Publication No. 1000, Series 3, No. 4, Oct. 1965.

International comparison of perinatal and infant mortality: The United States and six west European countries. *Vital and Health Statistics—Analytical Studies.* National Center for Health Statistics. U.S. Department of Health, Education, and Welfare. Public Health Service Publication No. 1000, Series 3, No. 6, March 1967.

JACOBSON, H. N., and REID, D. E.: High-risk pregnancy. II. A pattern of comprehensive maternal and child care. *New Eng J Med, 271:* 302, 1964.

Japan. Law No. 156 of 13 July, 1948, including amendments up to 21 April, 1960. Eugenic Protection Law. (Laws under the jurisdiction of Public Health Bureau. Ministry of Health and Welfare, July, 1964, p. 5). *Int Digest of Health Legislation,* 1965, vol. 16.

JAMES, G.: Poverty and public health—new outlooks. I. Poverty as an obstacle to health progress in our cities. *Amer J Public Health,* 55:1757, 1965.

JEFFRIES, J. E., (Ed.): The adolescent unwed mother. *Ross Round Table on Maternal and Child Nursing.* Columbus, Ross Laboratories, 1965.

JENKINS, W. W.: An experimental study of the relationship of legitimate and illegitimate birth status to school and personal social adjustment of Negro children. *Amer J Sociol 64:*169, 1958.

JOHNSON, C. S.: *Shadow of the Plantation.* Chicago, U. of Chicago, 1934.

JOHNSON, C. S.: *Growing Up in the Black Belt.* Negro youth in the rural south. Washington, D.C.; Amer. Council on Education, 1941.

JOHNSON, W. R., and SCHUTT, M.: Sex education attitudes of school administrators and school board members. *J Sch Health, 36:*64, 1966.

JONES, W. C.; MEYER, H. J., and BORGATTA, E. F.: Social and psychological factors in status decisions of unmarried mothers. *J Marriage Family,* 25:224, 1962.

JUDGE, J. G.: Casework with the unmarried mother in a family agency. *Social Casework,* 32:7, 1951.

KAMMERER, P. G.: *The Unmarried Mother.* Boston, Little, 1918.

KASANIN, J., and HANDSCHIN, S.: Psychodynamic factors in illegitimacy. *Amer J Orthopsychiat, 11:*66, 1941.

KAWI, A., and PASAMANICK, B.: The association of factors of pregnancy with reading disorders in childhood. *JAMA, 166:*1420–1423, 1958.

KELLY, G.: *Medico-Moral Problems.* St. Louis, The Catholic Hospital Association of the United States and Canada, 1967.

KELLEY, J. L.: The school and unmarried mothers. *Children, 10:*60, 1963.

KINCAID, J. C.: Social pathology of foetal and infant loss. *Brit Med J,* 1:1057, 1965.

KINSEY, A. C., et al.: *Sexual Behavior in the Human Male.* Philadelphia, Saunders, 1948.

KINSEY, A. C. Illegal Abortion in the United States. Presented at a conference on abortion sponsored by the Planned Parenthood Federation of America, Inc. at Harden House and the New York Academy of Medicine, April 1955.

KINSEY, A. C., et al.: *Sexual Behavior in the Human Female.* Philadelphia, Saunders, 1953.

KINSEY, A. C., and CALDERONE, M. S. (Ed.): *Abortion in the United States.* New York, Harper, 1958.

KIRKENDALL, L. A., and COX, H. M.: Starting a sex education program. *Children,* 14:136, 1967.

KLUCKHOLN, C.: Have there been discernible shifts in American values during the past generation? In Morrison E. (Ed.):*The American Style.* New York, Harper, 1958.

KNAPP, P.: The attitudes of Negro unmarried mothers toward illegitimacy. *Smith College Studies in Social Work,* 17:153, 1946, abstract of thesis.

KNAPP, P., and CAMBRIA, S. T.: The attitudes of Negro unmarried mothers toward illegitimacy. *Smith College Studies in Social Work,* 17:185, 1947.

KNOBLOCH, H., and PASAMANICK, B.: The relationship of race and socioeconomic status to development of motor behavior patterns in infancy. In Pasamanick, B. (Ed.) *Social Aspects of Psychiatry.* Amer. Psychiat. Assoc., Washington, D.C., 1959 (Regional Research Report No. 10).

KNOBLOCH, H., and PASAMANICK, B.: Environmental factors affecting human development before and after birth. *Pediatrics,* 26:210, 1960.

KNOBLOCH, H., and PASAMANICK, B.: Complications of Pregnancy and Mental Deficiency. Ment. Retard. Proc. 1st Internat. Cong. Ment. Retard., 1960, p. 182.

KNOBLOCH, H., and PASAMANICK, B.: Mental subnormality: medical progress, part I-III, *New Eng J Med,* 266:1046, 1092, 1155, 1962.

KNOBLOCH, H., and PASAMANICK, B.: Prospective studies on the epidemiology of reproductive casualty: methods, findings, and some implications. *Merrill-Palmer Quart,* 12:27, 1966.

KOLBLOVA, V.: Legal abortion in Czechoslovakia. *JAMA,* 196:371, 1966.

Koos, E. H.: *The Health of Regionville*. New York, Columbia, 1954.

KRANTZ, K.: Comments in: The adolescent unwed mother. In Jeffries, J. E. (Ed.): *Ross Round Table on Maternal and Child Nursing*. Columbus, Ross Laboratories, 1965.

KRONICK, J. C.: An assessment of research knowledge concerning the unmarried mother. *Res. Perspectives on the Unmarried Mother*. New York, The Child Welfare League of America, 1962, p. 17.

KUHLEA, R. G.: Adolescence. In Harris, C. (Ed.): *Encyclopedia of Educational Research*. New York, Macmillan, 1960, pp. 24–30.

KUTNER, B., and GORDON, G.: Seeking care for cancer. *J Health Hum Behav*, 2:171, 1961.

LADER, L.: *Abortion—The Tragic Myth*. New York, Bobbs, 1966, p. 70.

LANDIS, J. T.: Statement for the Asilomar Conference on the Teenage Parent, Sponsored by the Governor's Advisory Committee on Children and Youth, April 16–17, 1964.

LAWRENCE, R. A.: Rochester, N. Y. February, 1965. (unpublished survey).

LEHFELDT, H.: Willful exposure to unwanted pregnancy (WEUP). *Amer J Obstet Gynec*, 78:661, 1959.

LESSER, A. J.: Current Problems of Maternity Care. The first Jessie M. Bierman Annual Lecture in Maternal and Child Health, delivered May 10, 1963 at the School of Public Health, University of California, Berkeley. Washington, D.C., U. S. Department of Health, Education and Welfare, Welfare Administration, Children's Bureau, 1963.

LEVY, D.: A follow-up study of unmarried mothers. *Social Casework*, 36:27, 1955.

LILIENFELD, A. M.; PASAMANICK, B., and ROGERS, M. E.: The relationship between pregnancy experience and the development of certain neuropsychiatric disorders in childhood. *Amer J Public Health*, 45:637, 1955.

LIPSET, S. M.: *Political Man*. Garden City, Doubleday, 1960.

LOWE, C.: The intelligence and social background of the unmarried mother. *Ment Hyg*, 11:783, 1927.

LUCKEY, E. B.: Helping children grow up sexually. How, when, by whom? *Children*, 14:130, 1967.

LYONS, D. J.: Developing a Program for Pregnant Teen-agers Through the Cooperation of School, Health Department and Federal Agencies. Speech presented at a joint session of the American School Health Association and the American Public Health Association Annual Meeting, Miami Beach, Florida, October 24, 1967.

McClure, W. E.: Intelligence of unmarried mothers. *Psychol Clin,* 20:154, 1931.

McClure, W. E., and Goldberg, B.: Intelligence of unmarried mothers. *Psychol Clin, 18*:119, 1929.

McDonald, R. L., and Parham, K. J.: Relation of emotional changes during pregnancy to obstetric complications in unmarried primigravidas. *Amer J Obstet Gynec, 90*:195, 1964.

Mangold, G. B.: *Children Born Out of Wedlock.* Columbia, U. of Mo., 1921.

Marchetti, A. A., and Menaker, J. S.: Pregnancy and the adolescent. *Amer J Obstet Gynec, 59*:1013, 1950.

Maryland State Department of Education: *Pupil Drop-Out Study: Maryland Public High Schools, 1960–61.* April 1961.

May, R.: *The Meaning of Anxiety.* New York, Ronald, 1950.

Mayer, J.: The nutritional status of American Negroes. *Nutr Rev. 23:* 161, 1965.

Mead, M.: Lecture at Diablo Valley College, April 14, 1965.

Mead, M., and Wolfenstein, M. (Eds.): *Childhood in Contemporary Cultures.* Chicago, The U. of Chicago, 1955.

Mechanic, D., and Volkart, E. H.: Illness behavior and medical diagnoses. *J Health Hum Behav, 1*:89, 1960.

Mehlan, K. H.: Combating illegal abortion in the socialist countries of Europe. *World Med J, 13(3)*:84, 1966.

Meyer, H. J.; Jones, W., and Borgatta, E. F.: The decision of unmarried mothers to keep or surrender their babies. *Social Work, 1*:103, 1956.

Milman, D. H.: Adolescence: A subculture in United States society. *Bull NY Acad Med, 41*:347, 1965.

Model Penal Code, Sec. 207.11 (1957). *Cf.* text at note 57 *supra.*

Monahan, H. B., and Spender, E. C.: Deterrents to prenatal care. *Children, 9*:114, 1962.

Moriyama, I. M.: Present status of infant mortality problem in the United States. *Amer J Public Health, 56*:623, 1966.

Mussio, T. J.: Primigravidas under age 14. *Amer J Obstet Gynec, 84:* 442, 1962.

Myers, J. K., and Schaeffer, L.: Social stratification and psychiatric practice: A study of an outpatient clinic. *Amer Sociol Rev, 19:* 307, 1954.

Myrdal, G.: *An American Dilemma.* New York, Harper, 1944, pp. 177, 932.

Naegele, K. D.: Youth and society. Some observations. In Erikson,

E. H. (Ed.): *Youth: Change and Challenge.* New York, Basic Books, 1963, pp. 43–63.

National Office of Vital Statistics: *Vital Statistics of the United States 1958, Section 12,* General characteristics of live births. Washington, D.C., U.S. Department of Health, Education and Welfare, Public Health Service.

NESBITT, R. E. L., JR.: *Perinatal Loss in Modern Obstetrics.* Philadelphia, Davis, 1957.

NESBITT, R. E. L., JR.: Present Status of Maternal Health and Maternal Care. Problems in Perinatal Mortality and Morbidity. Pregnancy Wastage Programs. Primary Prevention from the Viewpoint of the Obstetrician. Proceedings, Bi-Regional Institute on Maternity Care—Primary Prevention. School of Public Health, University of California, Berkeley, June 21–25, 1964.

NESBITT, R. E. L., JR.; SCHLESINGER, R., and SHAPIRO, S.: Role of preventive medicine in reduction of infant and perinatal mortality. *Public Health Rep, 81:*691, 1966.

North Carolina General Statistics. 1967, Art. II, Chap. 14.

NORTH, A. F., JR.: Small-for-dates neonates. I. Maternal, gestational and neonatal characteristics. *Pediatrics, 38:*1013, 1966.

NOTTINGHAM, R. D. A psychological study of forty unmarried mothers. *Genet Psychol Monog, 19:*155, 1937.

ORNE, M. T.: On the social psychology of the psychological experiment—with particular reference to demand characteristics and their implications. *Amer Psychol, 17:*776, 1962.

ORNE, M. T., and EVANS, F. J.: Social control in the psychological experiment: Antisocial behavior and hypnosis. *J Personality Soc Psychol. 1:*189, 1965.

ORR, J. B., and PRILSIPHER, L.: *Education and Social Change.* Southwest Educational Development Laboratory, 1967, p. 159.

OSILI, A. J., and PARKER, F. A.: A follow-up study of fifty unmarried Negro mothers in active aid-to-dependent children cases in the Marion County Department of Public Welfare, Indianapolis, Indiana. Marion County Department of Public Welfare, January 24, 1967.

OSOFSKY, H. J.: Psychological and sociological issues in pregnancy. Presented at First Canadian National Conference on Maternal and Child Welfare, Ottawa, Canada, March 1967. *Med Serv J Canad, 23:*512, 1967.

OSOFSKY, H. J.: The Walls are Within (An exploration of barriers which interfere with the relationship between middle-class physicians and poor patients—with special emphasis upon the pregnant patient). In Deutscher, I., and Thompson, E. (Eds): *Among the People: Studies of the Urban Poor*. New York, Basic Books 1968c. (in press).

OSOFSKY, H. J.: Some social-psychological issues in improving obstetrical care for the poor. *Obstet Gynec, 31*:437, 1968d.

OSOFSKY, H. J.; HAGEN, J. H.; BRAEN, B. B.; WOOD, P. W., and DI-FLORIO, R.: Problems of the pregnant schoolgirl—an attempted solution. *NY J Med, 67*:2332, 1967a.

OSOFSKY, H. J.; HAGEN, J. H., and WOOD, P. W.: A program for pregnant schoolgirls—some early results. *Amer J Obstet Gynec, 100*:1020, 1968a.

OSOFSKY, H. J.; BRAEN, B.; DIFLORIO, R.; HAGEN, J. H., and WOOD, P. W.: A program for pregnant schoolgirls. A progress report. *Adolescence, 3*:89, 1968b.

OSTLUND, L. A.: Environment personality relationship. *Rural Sociol,* March, 1957.

PAKTER, J.; ROSNER, H. J.; JACOBZINER, H., and GREENSTEIN, F.: Out-of-wedlock births in New York City. I. Sociologic aspects. *Amer J Public Health, 51*:683, 1961a.

PAKTER, J.; ROSNER, H. J.; JACOBZINER, H., and GREENSTEIN, F.: Out-of-wedlock births in New York City. II. Medical aspects. *Amer J Public Health, 51*:846, 1961b.

PARSONS, T.: The school class as a social system—some of its functions in American society. *Harvard Ed Rev, 29(4)*: Fall, 1959, p. 297.

PARSONS, T.: Social change and medical organization in the United States: A sociological perspective. *Ann Amer Soc Political Social Sci, 346*:21, 1963.

PASAMANICK, B.: *The Epidemiology of Behavior Disorders of Childhood*. (Neurol. Psychiat. Childh. Res. Publ. Assoc. Nerv. Ment. Dis.) Baltimore, Williams & Wilkins, 1956.

PASAMANICK, B.; KNOBLOCH, H., and LILIENFIELD, A. M.: Socioeconomic status and some precursors of neuropsychiatric disorder. *Amer J Orthopsychiat, 26*:595, 1956.

PASAMANICK, B.: Research on the influence of sociocultural variables upon organic factors in mental retardation. *Amer J Ment Defic, 64*:316, 1959.

PASAMANICK, B., and KNOBLOCH, H.: Retrospective studies on the epidemiology of reproductive casualty: Old and new. *Merrill-Palmer Quart, 12*:7, 1966.

PATRIARCHE, M. E.: Sex education in the schools—the doctor's role. *Canad Med Ass J*, 96:377, 1967.

PAUL, B. D.: Anthropological perspectives on medicine and public health. *Ann Amer Soc Political Soc Sci*, 346:34, 1963.

PEARSON, J. S., and AMACHER, P. L.: Intelligence test results and observations of personality disorder among 3594 unwed mothers in Minnesota. *J Clin Psychol*, 12:16, 1956.

POLLIAKOFF, S. R.: Pregnancy in the young primigravida. *Amer J Obstet Gynec*, 76:746, 1958.

Population Profile—The Teen-age Mother. Washington, D.C., Population Reference Bureau, Inc., June 3, 1962.

POWDERMAKER, H.: *After Freedom: A Cultural Study in the Deep South*. New York, Viking, 1939, pp. 82, 160, 166.

POWELL, M.: Illegitimate pregnancy in emotionally disturbed girls. *Smith College Studies in Social Work*, 19:171, 1949.

(The) President's Panel on Mental Retardation: A Proposed Program for National Action to Combat Mental Retardation—Report to the President, October 1962. Washington, U.S. Government Printing Office, 1963.

PUTNOME, PETER (quoted in): If you had a choice, *Saturday Review* October 26, 1962, p. 53.

RANKIN, R. R.: Statement for the Asilomar Conference on the Teen-age Patient, Sponsored by the Governor's Advisory Committee on Children and Youth, April 16–17, 1964.

RASHBAUM, W.; REHR, H.; PANETH, J., and GREENBERG, M.: A Study of Extra-Marital Pregnancies at the Mount Sinai Hospital. New York, Departments of Obstetrics and Social Service, The Mount Sinai Hospital, June 1962.

RASHBAUM, W.; REHR, H.; PANETH, J., and GREENBERG, M.: Pregnancy in unmarried women, medical and social characteristics. *J Mt Sinai Hosp*, 30:33, 1963.

RASHBAUM, W.; REHR, H.; PANETH, J., and GREENBERG, M.: Use of social services by unmarried mothers. *Children*, 10:11, 1963.

REDLICH, F. C.; HOLLINGSHEAD, A. B.; and BELLIS, E.: Social class differences in attitudes toward psychiatry. *Amer J Orthopsychiat*, 25:60, 1955.

REED, R.: *The Illegitimate Family in New York City*. New York, Columbia, 1934.

REEDER, S. J., and REEDER, L. G.: Some correlates of prenatal care among low income wed and unwed women. *Amer J Obstet Gynec*, 90:1304, 1964.

REMMERS, H. H., and RADLER, D. H.: *The American Teen-ager,* Indianapolis, Bobbs, 1957.

Report of the National Advisory Commission on Civil Disorders. New York, Bantam, 1968.

Report of a WHO Expert Committee: Health problems of adolescence. *WHO Techn Rep Ser,* 1965, No. 308.

REYNOLDS, J.: Problems of Forty-Four Negro Unmarried Mothers in St. Louis, Missouri, March 1940–March 1941. Digest of master's dissertation presented at St. Louis University Graduate School, St. Louis, Mo.

RIDER, R. V.; TABACK, M., and KNOBLOCH, H.: Associations between premature births and socioeconomic status. *Amer J Public Health,* 45:1022, 1955.

ROBERTS, R. W., (Ed.): *The Unwed Mother.* New York, Harper, 1966, 270 pp.

RODMAN, H.: Marital relationships in a Trinidad village. *Marriage and Family Living,* 23:170, 1961.

RODMAN, H.: The lower-class value stretch. *Social Forces,* 42:205, 1963.

ROEMER, R.: Abortion law: The approaches of different nations. *Amer J Public Health,* 57:1906, 1967.

ROSE, A. M.: Reference groups of rural high school youth. *Child Develop,* 27:351, 1956.

ROSENTHAL, R.: On the social psychology of the psychological experiment. The experimenter's hypothesis as unintended determinant of experimental results. *Amer Sci,* 51:268, 1963.

ROSENTHAL, R.: Experimental outcome-orientation and the results of the psychological experiment. *Psychol Bull,* 61:405, 1964.

ROSENTHAL, R., and FODE, K. L.: Psychology of the scientist: V. Three experiments in experimenter bias. *Psychol Rep,* 12:491, 1963.

ROSENTHAL, R., and LAWSON, R.: A longitudinal study of the effects of experimenter bias on the operant learning of laboratory rats. *J Psychiat Res,* 2:61, 1963.

SARREL, P. M.: The university hospital and the teen-age unwed mother. *Amer J Public Health,* 57:1308, 1967.

SARREL, P. M., and DAVIS, C. D.: The young unwed primipara. A study of 100 cases with 5 year follow-up. *Amer J Obstet Gynec,* 95:722, 1966.

SARREL, P., Personal Communication, 1967.

SCHAUFFLER, G. D.: Maternity minus marriage. *Gen Pract,* 11:74, 1955.

SCHNIDEBERG, M.: Psychiatric-social factors in young unmarried mothers. *Social Casework, 32*:3, 1951.

SCHUMACHER, H. C.: The unmarried mother: A socio-psychiatric viewpoint. *Ment Hyg, 11*:775, 1927.

SELLTIZ, C., JAHODA, M., DEUTSCH, M., and COOK, S. W.: *Research Methods in Social Relations.* New York, Holt, 1959.

SEMMENS, J. P.: Implications in teen-age pregnancy. *Obstet Gynec, 26*:77, 1965.

SHAPIRO, S.; JACOBZINER, H.; DENSEN, P. M., WEINER, L.: Further observations on prematurity and perinatal mortality in a general population and in the population of a prepaid group practice medical care plan. *Amer J Public Health, 50*:1304, 1960.

SHAPIRO, S.; SCHLESINGER, E.; NESBITT, R. E. L., JR.: Infant and perinatal mortality in the United States. *Public Health Serv,* Oct. 1965.

SIECUS Newsletter, New York, Spring, 1965, Vol. 1, No. 1.

SIMMONS, O. G.: Implications of social class to public health. *Hum Organization, 16*:7, 1957.

SMITH, C. A.: Effects of maternal undernutrition upon the newborn infant in Holland (1944–1945). *J Pediat, 30*:229, 1947.

STEARN, R. H.: The adolescent primigravida. *Lancet, 2*:1083, 1963.

STINE, O. C.; RIDER, R. V., and SWEENEY, E.: School leaving due to pregnancy in an urban adolescent population. *Amer J Public Health, 54*:1, 1964.

SPIEGEL, L. A.: Comments on the psychoanalytic psychology of adolescence. *Psychoanalytic Study of the Child.* New York, Int. Univs., *13*:296, 1958.

STOCKWELL, E. G.: A critical examination of the relationship between socioeconomic status and mortality. *Amer J Public Health, 53*:956, 1963.

STONE, L. J., and CHURCH, J.: *Childhood and Adolescence* New York, Random, 1957.

SZASZ, T. S., and HOLLENDER, M. H.: A contribution of the philosophy of medicine. The basic models of the doctor-patient relationship. *Amer Med Ass Arch Int Med, 97*:585, 1956.

TAEUBER, K.: Negro residential segregation. Trends and measurement. *Social Problems, 12*:42, Summer, 1964.

TEELE, J. E.; ROBINSON, D.; SCHMIDT, W. M., and RICE, E. P.: Factors related to social work services for mothers of babies born out of wedlock. *Amer J Public Health 57*:1300, 1967.

Therapeutic Abortion Act. Calif. Sess. Laws 1967, ch. 327.

THOMPSON, J. D.: Improving Maternity Care. 1961, (unpublished).

THOMPSON, W. B.; MONTGOMERY, T. A., and REVENSCROFT, J. W.: California Maternal Mortality Survey, Study sponsored jointly by the California Medical Association and the State Department of Public Health, Berkeley, California, Aug. 1, 1957-Jan. 1, 1964, p. 6.

TIETZE, C.: Abortion in Europe. *Amer J Public Health,* 57:1923, 1967.

TOUSSIENG, P. W.: Psychosexual development in childhood and adolescence. *J Sch Health,* 35:158, 1965.

TUTTLE, E.: Serving the unwed mother who keeps her child. *Social Casework,* 43:415, 1962.

Unmarried mothers—and their children. Editorial, *Lancet,* 1:380, 1961.

Unmarried Mothers in the Municipal Court of Philadelphia. Philadelphia, Thomas Skelton Harrison Foundation, 1933.

Unmarried Parenthood—Clues to Agency and Community Action. New York, National Council on Illegitimacy, 1967.

VINCENT, C. E.: *Unmarried Mothers.* New York, Free Press of Glencoe, 1961.

VINCENT, C. E.: Unwed mother and sampling bias. *Amer Sociol Rev,* 19:562, 1954.

VINCENT, C. E.: Ego involvement in sexual relation: Implications for research on illegitimacy. *Amer J Sociol,* 65:287, 1959.

VINCENT, C. E.: Unmarried fathers and the mores: Sexual exploiter as an ex post facto label. *Amer Sociol Rev,* 25:40, 1960.

VINCENT, C. E.: Unwed mothers and the adoption market. Psychological and familial factors. *Marriage and Family Living,* 22:112, 1960.

WALLACE, H. M.: Teen-age pregnancy. *Amer J Obstet Gynec,* 92:1125, 1965.

WARKANY, J.: Congenital malformations induced by maternal nutritional deficiency. *J Pediat,* 25:476, 1944.

WATTS, L. G., *et al.*: *The Middle-Income Negro Family Faces Urban Renewal.* Waltham, Mass., Brandeis University, 1964, p. 44, 54, 60, 68.

WEBB, E. J.; CAMPBELL, D. T.; SCHWARTZ, R. D., and SECHREST, L.: *Unobtrusive Measures: Nonreactive Research in the Social Sciences.* Chicago, Rand McNally, 1966.

Welfare Law Bulletin, January 1968, No. 11, p. 10.

WELLIN, E.: Implications of local culture for public health, *Hum Organization 16*:16, 1958.

WHITEMAN, M., BROWN, B. and DEUTSCH, M. Some Effects of Social Class and Race on Children's Language and Intellectual Abilities. In

Deutsch, M. (Ed.): *The Disadvantaged Child.* New York, Basic Books, Inc., 1967, pp. 319–335.

WHITING, J. W. M., and CHILD, I. L.: *Child Training and Personality: A Cross Cultural Study.* New Haven, Yale, 1953.

WILLIAMS, G.: Euthanasia and abortion. *Univ Colorado Law Rev,* 38:178, 194, 1966.

WILTSE, K. T., and ROBERTS, R. W.: Illegitimacy and the AFDC Program. In Roberts, R. W. (Ed.): *The Unwed Mother.* New York, Harper, 1966, pp. 218–230.

WRIGHT, M. K.: Comprehensive services for adolescent unwed mothers. *Children, 13*:171, 1966.

YOUNG, L. R.: *Out of Wedlock.* New York, McGraw, 1960.

YOUNG, L. R.: Personality patterns in unmarried mothers. *The Family,* 1945, Vol. 26, No. 8.

YOUNG, L. R.: The unmarried mother: Problems of financial support. *Social Casework, 35*:99, 1954.

INDEX